The Quick and Easy
Sleep Apnea
Book

The Quick and Easy
Sleep Apnea
Book

Gautam Soparkar, MD

Library of Congress Control Number: 2010910990
ISBN: Hardcover   978-1-4535-4585-0
                  Softcover   978-1-4535-4584-3
                  Ebook   978-1-4535-4586-7

This book was printed in the United States of America.

Diagrams by:

Mihir Soparkar
Gautam Soparkar

To order additional copies of this book, contact:
Xlibris Corporation
1-888-795-4274
www.Xlibris.com
Orders@Xlibris.com
74657

Contents

To my late parents, Anjani and Ramesh Soparkar;
my late mother-in-law, Manjula Narayanan;
and my father-in-law, K. M. Narayanan.

. . . on the box sat a fat and red-faced boy, in a state of somnolency . . .

. . . "Damn that boy," said the old gentleman, "he's gone to sleep again."

"Very extraordinary boy, that," said Mr. Pickwick; "does he always sleep in this way?"

"Sleep!" said the old gentleman, "he's always asleep. Goes on errands fast asleep, and snores as he waits at table."

(From *The Posthumous Papers of the Pickwick Club*
(The Pickwick Papers)
by Charles Dickens, 1837)

Disclaimer

The information contained in this book is not intended to replace professional healthcare advice, or to be a means of self-diagnosis or self-treatment. It is also not meant to be an exhaustive source of information. Readers are advised to discuss any health problem or treatment they may require with a qualified healthcare provider.

The author and publisher will not be responsible for any losses, injuries, illnesses, or damages arising, either directly or indirectly, from the use of the information contained in this book.

Foreword

If you are reading this, you probably have sleep apnea, think you might have it, or know someone who might have it. If not, you may just be interested in knowing more about an important medical condition that is becoming more common yet remains relatively unknown. Either way, this book is for you.

There are many excellent books on sleep disorders, but most of them deal with sleep problems as a whole. As a result, if you want information about something specific like sleep apnea, you will generally find it associated or combined with other information that is not relevant. For example, sleep apnea may be discussed with insomnia, which is not the same condition, although both are important sleep-related issues. I believe if you are looking for something specific, you should not have to sift through mountains of information to find it.

It is also increasingly clear that you cannot think of sleep apnea in isolation, because it is now known to be the cause of, or is associated with, many other medical problems. High blood pressure (hypertension) and heart disease are just some of the conditions that have been closely linked to sleep apnea. It is obvious that this condition is no longer the exclusive domain of "sleep specialists" or "sleep medicine" but figures in the treatment of many people who see their health care providers for other reasons.

This book has been written to provide information as well as to dispel some of the misconceptions about sleep apnea. The book can be read

14   GAUTAM SOPARKAR, MD

either from beginning to end or as individual chapters, which I have tried to make as "stand-alone" as possible. The last chapter consists of frequently asked questions. Some of the questions and also some of the diagrams are adapted from my previous book, *Questions and Answers in Sleep Apnea (An Internist's Perspective)*, published by Xlibris. Most chapters are followed by key points under the heading "At a Glance" for easy review.

I am indebted to my patients, whose management has been extremely rewarding and a continuing source of personal learning. Thanks are also due to my colleagues for their support and advice. Much of the material was gathered by reading around my patients, informal discussions with colleagues, and so-called corridor consultations, the value of which cannot be overestimated. I would also like to acknowledge the support of the staff at the Bluewater Sleep Disorder Clinic, Sarnia, and the Leamington Sleep Clinic, Leamington. I am grateful to my wife, Arati, and daughter, Samira, for their unflagging patience and support. Special thanks are due to my son, Mihir, for his help with the diagrams.

I have included some material that is not readily available in other places. Information about other sleep disorders has been largely omitted. The concise approach will hopefully be informative, readily accessible, and useful without producing an information overload. The challenge has been to keep this book short as well as informative. Details of the physiology of sleep apnea have been kept to a minimum. These can be found in greater detail in other sources of reference, a selection of which appears in the bibliography, which includes medical textbooks, other books meant for general readership, and useful web sites.

I have tried to maintain a balanced approach to the description, diagnosis, and treatment of sleep apnea, keeping controversies to a minimum. Nevertheless, it must be recognized that there is always an alternate point of view, and not everyone will agree with certain statements in the text. Omissions are inevitable due to the compact size of the book. Every effort has been made to ensure accuracy, but some errors may have crept in, for which I am solely responsible.

Suggestions and comments are welcome and may be sent to *soparkar1@gmail.com.*

Gautam Soparkar, MBBS, DTCD, MD, MRCP(UK), FRCPC
Internist and Pulmonologist
Adjunct Professor of Medicine
Preceptor, Southwestern Ontario Medical Education Network
Schulich School of Medicine and Dentistry, University of Western Ontario
London, Ontario, Canada

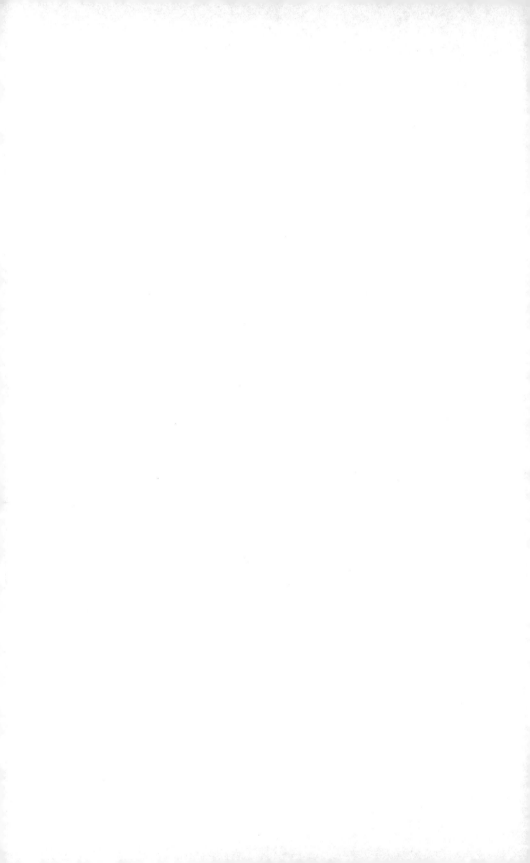

Abbreviations

ADHD: attention deficit hyperactivity disorder
AHI: apnea-hypopnea index
ANP: atrial natriuretic peptide
ASV: adaptive servo-ventilation
BiPAP: bilevel positive airway pressure
BMI: body mass index
CBT: cognitive behavior therapy
CHF: congestive heart failure
COPD: chronic obstructive pulmonary disease
CPAP: continuous positive airway pressure
CSA: central sleep apnea
EKG: electrocardiogram
ENT: ear, nose, and throat
OHS: obesity-hypoventilation syndrome
OSA: obstructive sleep apnea
OSAHS: obstructive sleep apnea hypopnea syndrome
OSAS: obstructive sleep apnea syndrome
PAH: pulmonary artery hypertension
PSG: polysomnogram
RDI: respiratory disturbance index
REM: rapid eye movement
RERA: respiratory effort-related arousal
SDB: sleep-disordered breathing
UARS: upper airway resistance syndrome
UPPP: uvulopalatopharyngoplasty

Chapter 1

Introduction

Take a look at the following scenarios:

1. A sixty-year-old overweight man who is recovering from a heart attack.
2. A twelve-year-old boy who is not doing well at school.
3. A thirty-year-old woman who is seven months pregnant and feeling extremely tired.
4. A fifty-year-old woman who has recently gained weight and is being treated (unsuccessfully) for depression.

What is the common factor? At first glance, it might appear that these four individuals have nothing in common, except perhaps that all of them may have some health issues. However, if you knew that each of them snores loudly and is very sleepy during the day, the answer would be *sleep apnea*. The point here is that sleep apnea can show up in different situations and in many ways. This is a condition that has only recently emerged as a major health problem, and even so, its full significance in the general population is not well recognized.

Sleep apnea literally means "cessation of breathing during sleep" (Greek: *apnea* = without breath). Descriptions of sleep apnea or its variations are actually quite old, having been found in several ancient texts.

The East Indian epic *Ramayana* mentions Kumbhakarna, brother of the emperor of Lanka (modern Sri Lanka). According to the narrative,

Kumbhakarna slept for six months at a time; and while he was asleep, he snored loudly and was hard to rouse. He had a voracious appetite when he was awake and was very obese, presumably from compulsive eating. "Ondine's curse" is the name given to a particular type of sleep apnea and comes from European mythology, according to which Ondine, a water nymph, cursed her unfaithful lover so that he would stop breathing if he fell asleep. Other references to what we now know as sleep apnea can be found in various other ancient works.

The first modern, albeit unwitting, reference to sleep apnea can probably be credited to Charles Dickens in *The Pickwick Papers*, published in the early nineteenth century. There can be no mistaking the classic features of sleep apnea in the combination of obesity, snoring, and sleepiness attributed to the boy Joe, although the health implications were likely not appreciated at the time. The term "Pickwickian syndrome" was coined later to describe an extreme form of sleep apnea that combines obesity, snoring, pauses in breathing, daytime sleepiness, and shallow breathing even while awake. In this condition, the carbon dioxide level in the blood is usually high, producing the red face described by Dickens.

With so many past references to snoring, obesity, sleepiness, and other features, it seems incredible that sleep apnea was generally not considered a medical problem until well into the twentieth century. Even when sleep apnea was described in the medical literature in 1956 by Burwell, it was little more than an interesting phenomenon; apart from a few committed researchers, not many people were interested in the subject.

It is only in the last twenty to thirty years that sleep apnea has received attention as a major health problem, not only because of its effect on sleep quality, but also because it can lead to many other health conditions. Sleep apnea also commonly occurs along with other medical conditions without necessarily causing them. These conditions are described in this book, either under consequences of sleep apnea (chapter 4) or under sleep apnea and special situations (chapter 8). The scenarios mentioned at the beginning of this chapter partly illustrate this point, and the connections will hopefully become clearer as you go through the book.

It is now possible to investigate and treat this increasingly common condition effectively. If you have sleep apnea, think you might have it, or know someone who does, read on.

At a Glance:

- Descriptions of sleep apnea or its variations are quite old, having been found in ancient mythological texts.
- Sleep apnea can show up in diverse situations.
- Sleep apnea has only recently been recognized as an important medical condition. Even so, its full significance is not generally appreciated.

Chapter 2

What Is Sleep Apnea?

Sleep apnea is a condition in which a person stops breathing, either completely or partially, over and over again during sleep. These interruptions in breathing can be several seconds or even minutes long. The pauses in breathing disturb the normal sleep pattern and, if they are long enough, drop the oxygen level in the blood.

Actually, sleep apnea is not a single condition. There are two main types: *obstructive* and *central* sleep apnea. A third type called "*mixed* sleep apnea" has the same causes, risk factors, and symptoms as obstructive apnea. The treatment of mixed apnea is also similar to that of obstructive apnea. For our purposes, therefore, we will consider mixed apnea a type of obstructive sleep apnea.

About 90 percent of sleep apnea is of the obstructive type, with central sleep apnea accounting for only about 10 percent. When the term "sleep apnea" is used, it usually refers to the obstructive type. This book deals mainly with obstructive sleep apnea, although some information about central sleep apnea is included in this and subsequent chapters.

In obstructive sleep apnea (OSA), the person is essentially strangled repeatedly during sleep. To picture this, think of the upper air passage (the part between the back of the nose and the voice-box or larynx) as a floppy rubber tube. Now imagine this rubber tube being repeatedly narrowed or closed off by negative pressure as the air inside is sucked out again and again. Something very similar happens to the air passage when a person has OSA.

In real life, the negative pressure occurs when the sleeping person breathes in, and the air passage closes off because the muscles holding it open are less active during sleep. Additionally, fatty tissue on the outside of the "tube" can narrow the passage, making it easier to get blocked. Large tonsils (inside the throat on either side) or adenoids (behind the nose in the air passage) or a large tongue can also make the obstruction worse from inside the "tube." The end result is repeated narrowing and collapse of the air passage, which prevents air from going into the lungs.

When the air passage closes off, the person struggles to breathe and wakes up (usually just partially, sometimes fully), and the muscles which maintain the patency of the air passage become more active. The obstruction is then relieved, and normal breathing resumes, allowing the person to fall asleep again. This happens over and over again during the night, resulting in recurrent mechanical blockage of the upper air passage and interruption of breathing.

Many of us have observed a sleeping person who snores loudly, then becomes quiet, then starts breathing again with a gasp or snort. This is the typical description of a person with OSA. If severe enough, the repeated partial or complete awakenings can result in non-restful sleep; and the pauses in breathing can drop the oxygen level in the blood, eventually leading to other medical problems.

The second and much less common type of sleep apnea is central sleep apnea (CSA) in which there are pauses in breathing during sleep without obstruction to the air passage. In this case, the brain "forgets" to send signals to the lungs to breathe. Since blockage of the air passage is not required to produce CSA, snoring is usually not a major symptom and may not be present at all (unless OSA is also present—both types can occur in the same person). CSA is often the result of other medical conditions like some brain disorders or heart failure or because of drugs like sleeping pills or narcotics that suppress brain activity.

Figure 1 shows the difference between obstructive and central apnea. In both cases, there is no flow of air (apnea). In OSA, the muscles of breathing continue to work to try to breathe; whereas in CSA, there is no effort from the muscles of breathing because they are not receiving the right signals from the brain.

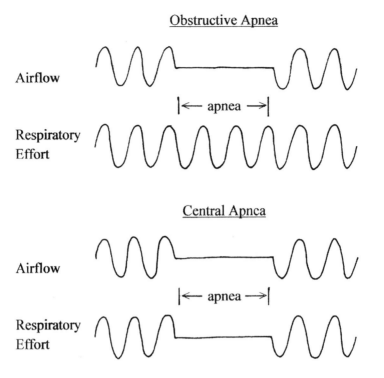

Figure 1. Difference between obstructive and central sleep apnea
[Adapted from: *Questions and Answers in Sleep Apnea (An Internist's Perspective)*
by Gautam Soparkar, Xlibris, 2009]

Both OSA and CSA can occur in the same person. When this happens, OSA is usually more severe than CSA. One can suspect OSA and CSA from symptoms and by watching a sleeping person, but to really tell them apart and to know their severity, you need a sleep study (chapter 5).

At a Glance:

- Sleep apnea is a condition in which a person stops (or comes close to stopping) breathing many times in a night.
- Sleep apnea is of two main types—obstructive (OSA) and central (CSA).
- Obstructive sleep apnea (OSA) is the most common type (about 90 percent) in which the upper air passage closes off (completely or partially) during sleep, producing obstruction to the passage of air.
- Central sleep apnea (CSA) is much less common (about 10 percent). In this condition, the brain "forgets" to tell the lungs to breathe. It is often a result of other medical conditions or certain medications.

Chapter 3

Snoring and Sleep Apnea: Making the Connection

We all know people who snore, sometimes very loudly. We may even recognize ourselves or a family member as being among them. Sleep apnea goes hand in hand with snoring, but they are not the same thing.

Snoring is the noise made by air as it passes in and out through the upper air passage, making the uvula and soft palate vibrate in the throat. Some people think you can snore only with your mouth open: this is not true since the vibrations can occur even with a closed mouth while the person is breathing through the nose. Partially blocked nasal passages can also cause snoring; in that case, the sound comes from the nose.

Sleep apnea is stoppage or near-stoppage of breathing during sleep. Partial interruption of breathing can occur at the same time as snoring since some air can get through, but complete stoppage of breathing can only occur *in between* periods of snoring.

The vast majority of people who have sleep apnea, especially OSA, also snore; it is very unusual for sleep apnea to be present without snoring. The converse is not true—snorers do not necessarily have sleep apnea. Snoring without sleep apnea is called "primary" or "simple" snoring.

Both snoring and sleep apnea occur because of excessive floppiness or narrowing of the upper air passage. This is more common in people who are overweight or obese, have a thick neck, or (less commonly) have certain anatomical features, such as a recessed chin. Overweight and obese individuals tend to snore more often and louder than people of normal weight; they are also more likely to have sleep apnea. Most people who have sleep apnea are overweight or obese, although this condition can be seen even in non-obese persons. By itself, snoring is little more than an annoyance to other people and often a source of amusement. However, when it is associated with sleep apnea, it needs to be taken more seriously.

Snoring is very common. The actual numbers vary from study to study, but according to one source, 40 percent of men and 24 percent of women snore (with or without sleep apnea). In fact, snoring is so common that it is a part of life for many people, their spouses, and families. Stories depict snoring as being associated with deep and restful sleep for the sleeper (though not for the person who has to listen to it!), but this is not really true. Snoring can be a sign that sleep apnea may also be present, particularly when it is loud or combined with gasping breaths. In summary, snoring and sleep apnea are two different but closely related conditions that commonly occur together, with snoring being a "red flag" for sleep apnea.

Sleep apnea is also very common, though not as much as snoring. The problem is that many people with sleep apnea do not have any symptoms (other than snoring, which is usually noticed by someone else). Count the number of people who have sleep apnea *with symptoms,* and about 4 percent of men and 2 percent of women will qualify. If you include people who have sleep apnea, *with or without symptoms*, the numbers jump to about 24 percent of men and 9 percent of women. Take away the people who have symptoms, and you get about 20 percent of men and 7 percent of women with sleep apnea *but no symptoms*. These are very approximate numbers but, nevertheless, indicate firstly that sleep apnea is very common and secondly, that most people with this condition have no symptoms and are probably unaware they have it.

The muscles holding the upper air passage open become more lax with age. Also, weight gain is more common as people get older. Older persons are also more likely to take more medications, some of which worsen sleep apnea, for example sleeping pills and certain painkillers. For these reasons, sleep apnea tends to become more common as people get older.

Remarkably, although sleep apnea is so common, information about it is not. Ask people what diabetes is, and most of them will know about it. Ask the same people what sleep apnea is, and chances are they will either not know or will be misinformed about it. Even many people in the health care field do not know much about sleep apnea because most of the research and information is very recent. Sleep-related disorders in general and sleep apnea in particular were not part of the general medical curriculum a couple of decades ago. Even now, these subjects are not well taught in medical schools.

Like the condition itself, misinformation about sleep apnea is common. A lot of this comes from word of mouth or from well-meaning but not-so-well-informed health advocates. Many people do not know about sleep apnea or think it means just not sleeping well. Examples of such misinformation include believing that sleep apnea and insomnia are the same (they are not) and that there is only one way to treat sleep apnea (actually, there are many ways, though some are better than others). Some people think they sleep well and can't possibly have sleep apnea because they fall asleep before their head hits the pillow. Actually, this is a sign of excessive sleepiness, which can be caused by sleep apnea!

Figure 2 indicates the approximate percentage of men and women who snore, those who have sleep apnea without symptoms and those who have sleep apnea with symptoms. In all categories, men are affected more often than women, though these are by no means "men's" conditions.

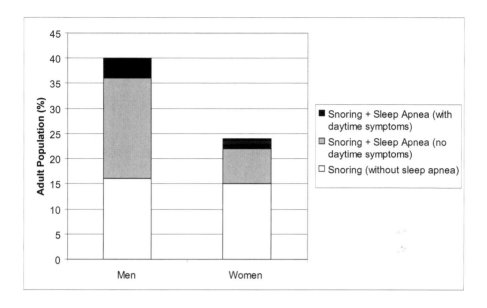

Figure 2. Snoring and sleep apnea in men and women

Recent studies have shown that the risk of sleep apnea in women increases after menopause.

There is a marked lack of awareness that untreated sleep apnea, especially if it is severe, can lead to other potentially serious medical problems. As a result, sleep apnea is not taken seriously by a lot of people who might benefit from good treatment, sometimes until it is too late.

Most people who have this condition are not aware of it. It is a sobering thought that at least three out of four people with *severe* sleep apnea don't even know they have a condition that is potentially lethal! This is very unfortunate, especially since sleep apnea is eminently treatable.

At a Glance:

- Snoring is a "red flag" for sleep apnea, especially if it is loud. The vast majority of people with sleep apnea also snore, but many snorers do not have sleep apnea.
- Both snoring and sleep apnea are more common in overweight or obese people. A narrow and floppy upper air passage is the common factor responsible for both.
- Most, but not all, people with sleep apnea are overweight or obese.
- Awareness about sleep apnea is lacking, and there is a lot of misinformation.
- Most people with sleep apnea don't even know they have it.

Chapter 4

Consequences of Sleep Apnea

Sleep apnea affects people in two ways: directly due to poor sleep quality and because of medical conditions that can develop later if it remains untreated.

The results of poor sleep quality are similar to what happens if someone is sleep-deprived for other reasons. Excessive sleepiness, tiredness, lack of concentration, and irritability are familiar to anyone who has not slept well for even a night or two. More subtle changes in memory or personality can also be seen. Other problems include moodiness and even impotence. Sometimes the symptoms are mistaken for depression or chronic fatigue syndrome. With sleep apnea, headaches can occur first thing in the morning due to accumulation of carbon dioxide in the blood; typically, the headaches disappear within an hour or so when the person begins to breathe better after waking up.

Excessive daytime sleepiness has received a lot of attention, particularly since it can lead to accidents. It is of particular concern in occupations that require a high degree of alertness, such as airline pilots or long-distance truck drivers. Even people who think they are not sleepy may suffer from so-called microsleeps. These are extra-short episodes of sleep that last just seconds, usually without the person being aware of them. The very brief loss of awareness of the surroundings can be devastating in situations that demand constant alertness, such as driving. A driver who has such microsleeps is sometimes jolted awake when the tires hit the "rumble strips" on the edge of the freeway: this is a warning that the person is very sleepy and needs to pull over for a short nap!

Sleepiness and tiredness (or fatigue), are not the same. You may be tired after running a marathon, but not necessarily sleepy. If you stay up late at night, you may be sleepy the next day, but not necessarily tired. Sleepiness is an overwhelming urge to sleep—such a person will fall asleep within minutes or even seconds if allowed to do so (a person who is not unduly sleepy normally takes ten minutes or longer to fall asleep). Some sleepy people will have microsleeps as described above without actually realizing they are sleepy. Tiredness, on the other hand, is a feeling of exhaustion, sometimes described as feeling "drained" or "wiped out."

People who are tired but not sleepy know the feeling of lying down, feeling exhausted, but not being able to fall asleep. Of course, sleepiness and tiredness can occur together, which may be why many people think they are the same.

It is important to remember that sleepiness, fatigue, and many of the symptoms mentioned above are not seen only with sleep apnea but also in other situations. For example, insufficient sleep can also cause sleepiness; if this is the case, the answer is to get more sleep. Similarly, sleep that is not restful because of some type of pain requires treatment of whatever is causing the pain. In other words, excessive daytime sleepiness and other daytime symptoms do not necessarily mean a person has sleep apnea, but are just an indication that something may be wrong with the quality or duration of sleep at night.

Many simple methods have been developed to help people find out if they need to be checked for sleep apnea. For example, the American Sleep Apnea Association has the so-called snore score questionnaire on its web site (www.sleepapnea.org). This includes six questions:

1. Are you a loud and/or regular snorer?
2. Have you ever been observed to gasp or stop breathing during sleep?
3. Do you feel tired or groggy upon awakening, or do you awaken with a headache?

4. Are you often tired or fatigued during the wake-time hours?
5. Do you fall asleep sitting, reading, watching TV, or driving?
6. Do you often have problems with memory or concentration?

Obviously, there are many reasons for having these symptoms, but a "yes" answer to one or more of these questions increases the chances of having sleep apnea, especially if one is also overweight. Other similar questionnaires have been developed, inquiring about symptoms that might point to sleep apnea, although no questionnaire can confirm sleep apnea without further testing.

Some symptoms of central sleep apnea (CSA) are similar to those of obstructive sleep apnea (OSA), such as sleepiness and tiredness, because sleep is disrupted in both cases. In addition, there may be symptoms of the underlying medical problem responsible for the CSA. For example, the person may show signs of paralysis or speech defects if a stroke has caused the CSA or may be very short of breath and unable to lie flat if heart failure is present.

The initial suspicion that a person might have sleep apnea often comes from observations made by someone else. Loud snoring, gasping breaths during sleep, or actual pauses in breathing are usually noticed by the sleep partner. At other times, the affected person notices daytime symptoms such as sleepiness or fatigue, which are the result of not getting restful sleep. Occasionally, sleep apnea comes to light in other ways; for example, when a person is hospitalized for an unrelated illness and healthcare staff notice the symptoms, or when a person receives a general anesthetic, which can bring out the signs and symptoms of sleep apnea.

Sleep partners or family members of people with sleep apnea often report that the person becomes silent between periods of snoring. These silent periods may be normal breaths but may also be pauses in breathing between the snoring episodes, i.e., apneas. Although snoring is unmistakable, it takes a very observant person to notice pauses in breathing, which is why people are often surprised when sleep studies show the number of pauses—sometimes this happens over a hundred times an hour! This is also one reason why you can't tell the severity of sleep apnea just by watching a sleeping person; for this, you need a sleep study.

Untreated sleep apnea can also lead to other medical conditions, especially if the sleep apnea is severe. The most important of these are high blood pressure (hypertension), coronary artery disease (narrowing of the arteries of the heart), and strokes. Together, they can be grouped under the category of *cardiovascular disease.*

Of all the links between sleep apnea and various conditions, the association with high blood pressure (hypertension) is the best known. About half of those with untreated sleep apnea have high blood pressure, and about a third of all people with hypertension have sleep apnea. Hypertension is usually "silent," with no symptoms initially—it is usually found when the blood pressure is measured routinely. Sleep apnea can make it difficult to control blood pressure, and this is sometimes the clue that leads to being tested for apnea. When the apnea is treated properly, the blood pressure often becomes easier to control and may even require less medication.

Sleep apnea also increases the risk of narrowing of the arteries, which in turn raises the risk of heart disease and stroke. Heart disease can show up as chest pain (especially on exertion, called angina), shortness of breath, or an actual heart attack. Sometimes it shows up as an abnormal heart rhythm (arrhythmia). A stroke may show up as a dramatic event like paralysis on one side of the body or with more subtle signs like some slurring of speech.

If any of these conditions develops in someone with sleep apnea, signs and symptoms of that particular condition may become obvious in addition to those already present from the apnea. In fact, the presence of these medical conditions should raise the possibility that sleep apnea might be present, regardless of whether or not there are symptoms directly from the apnea.

What is the connection between sleep apnea and these conditions? To understand this, we need to explore what actually happens during sleep when a person has apnea.

During sleep, in people without sleep apnea, the breathing becomes slightly shallow and the blood oxygen level drops very slightly. This is a normal occurrence and not a cause for alarm. With sleep apnea, there are major pauses in breathing (complete or near-complete), producing greater drops in the oxygen level, especially if the pauses are long. During the pauses, which are due to obstruction of the airway, the person struggles to breathe through a partially or totally blocked air passage until they manage to force it open and start breathing again with a snort or gasp, usually arousing partially from a deeper to a lighter stage of sleep.

The more severe the apnea, the more often this happens and the lower the oxygen level drops. In people with severe apnea, this can happen hundreds of times a night and literally millions of times over several years, putting a strain on the heart. With the repeated dips in oxygen level and the struggle to breathe, the body produces the so-called fight-or-flight substances, which raise blood pressure and increase the heart rate. Adrenaline is one such substance. Essentially, the body gets an "adrenaline rush" with every interruption in breathing.

Our hearts and arteries were not designed to take this kind of repeated buffeting. It is believed that over time, the repeated drops in oxygen level and the chemicals produced can permanently raise the blood pressure (hypertension). It can also narrow the arteries of the heart and brain, leading to heart attacks and strokes. Low oxygen levels by themselves can give rise to arrhythmias. A particular type of arrhythmia called *atrial fibrillation* can itself increase the chances of having a stroke.

Many of these conditions are more common in overweight or obese people anyway. If sleep apnea is also present, the risk is higher and the more severe the apnea, the greater the health risk.

All these conditions are related to each other in a very complex way (Figure 3). Weight gain by itself increases the risk of hypertension, heart problems, and strokes. Hypertension itself increases the risk of strokes and heart problems. Thus, one problem can lead to (or increase the risk of) another; and two or more conditions can be present at the same time, with one often reinforcing the other.

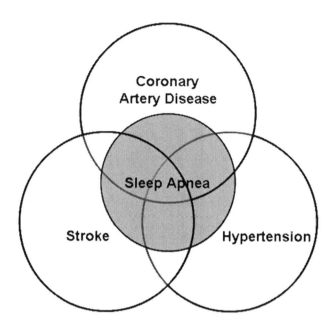

Figure 3. Sleep apnea and some related health problems

There also seems to be an increased risk of type 2 diabetes mellitus (the most common type) with sleep apnea and not just because of obesity, i.e., sleep apnea independently increases the risk of diabetes. The combination of obesity, high blood pressure, high cholesterol (particularly the "bad" cholesterol) and high blood sugar is known as the "metabolic syndrome": another indication that many of these conditions are interrelated and tend to occur together in the same person.

Sleep apnea can sometimes produce symptoms that seem completely unrelated, but there is usually an explanation. Acid reflux (which causes heartburn) is common in patients with sleep apnea, firstly because they are usually overweight, and excess weight itself can cause this problem. As well, acid from the stomach can be forced into the esophagus (the passage connecting the mouth to the stomach) when the person struggles to breathe because of sleep apnea. Sometimes a chemical called atrial natriuretic peptide (ANP) is produced in excess in the heart because of the stress of sleep apnea. This chemical makes a person produce more urine, requiring frequent visits to the washroom at night. The heartburn from acid reflux and repeated awakening to go to the washroom add to the sleep disruption produced by the sleep apnea itself.

An underactive thyroid gland (hypothyroidism) can indirectly produce sleep apnea by causing a person to put on weight. Some of the symptoms of an underactive thyroid, such as sleepiness and tiredness, are themselves very similar to those caused by sleep apnea. A simple blood test can identify an underactive thyroid gland, which can then be easily treated with thyroid hormone pills.

Sleep apnea has been reported to cause attacks of gout, a painful joint condition caused by increase in a substance called uric acid in the blood. Uric acid is the result of cell damage, which can occur because of low oxygen levels caused by sleep apnea.

Often, sleep apnea is suspected *after* a medical condition like heart disease or hypertension is diagnosed. People are commonly referred to sleep laboratories after having been found to have one of these conditions, and many people have found out they have sleep apnea after having a heart attack or after their blood pressure has been high for many years. Going back in the history of these people, it often turns out they had been overweight, snoring, and sleepy for years, but nobody had thought of sleep apnea simply because these symptoms are so easy to pass off.

Why should sleep apnea be treated? This is practically a no-brainer if sleep apnea is obviously affecting one's life and well-being. There are very few other conditions that are present only during sleep, but have such a profound effect on a person during waking hours. Sleep apnea can result in non-restful sleep, so much so that it can become impossible to even get through the day because of sleepiness and fatigue, let alone be productive and efficient. Treatment in such a situation can literally transform one's life.

If someone has sleep apnea, he or she may not be getting restful sleep. Often, the person complains of sleeping throughout the night yet feeling tired upon waking up. The ultimate result is the same as what would happen if he or she got very few hours of sleep. Sleep that is not restful produces excessive daytime sleepiness, lack of concentration, and moodiness. Many people don't realize the effect sleep apnea has on their alertness and concentration—it becomes obvious only when it is treated. This is like people who are short-sighted and need glasses for the first time. Sometimes they are themselves not aware of the reduction in their vision since it usually happens gradually. Once they get their vision tested and begin to use their glasses, they begin to see a whole new world and wonder how they managed earlier.

Depending upon how severe the condition is and also how well a person can cope, sleep apnea can affect day-to-day functioning. This is particularly important for people whose work requires a high level of concentration and alertness, such as long-distance drivers and airline pilots. Effective treatment generally results in dramatic improvement in symptoms. The more severe the symptoms, the more dramatic seems to be the improvement with treatment, especially with the technique of continuous positive airway pressure, or CPAP (see chapter 7). Many people say they have got their life back once sleep apnea is treated properly.

It is more of a hard sell to treat sleep apnea if a person has few or no symptoms. This is not uncommon since many people seem to cope with apnea quite well. For them, sleep apnea is not an issue; they are not aware of it and don't seem to feel the effects. Sleep apnea usually creeps up on people over years, and they may not even be aware of how much it is affecting their life and functioning. For such people, it is important to understand that there is another compelling reason to treat sleep apnea: the increased risk of developing the medical conditions mentioned above.

An additional, and often underrated, benefit of treating sleep apnea is the value to the sleep partner. When sleep apnea is treated, so is the snoring. Sleep partners of people with sleep apnea often spend troubled and restless nights themselves, disturbed by snoring and worrying about their partners. People who have previously been kept awake by their partners' snoring, or even had to sleep in separate rooms, find that when the apnea is treated, they are able to return to their bedrooms. They can then sleep without the disturbance of snoring or the stress of worrying about their partners' apnea!

In summary, finding and treating sleep apnea is helpful in many ways. Often, there are immediate benefits in terms of improved symptoms and feeling better, and this is a big motivating factor to continue treatment. At other times, the value of treating sleep apnea is not obvious immediately, but is likely to show over time. In such cases, it is important to remember to continue treatment even if one feels no benefit immediately. It is like treating high cholesterol, where treating it can improve a person's risk of heart attacks, strokes, and other problems in the long term, even if short-term benefits are not obvious.

At a Glance:

- Untreated sleep apnea can produce nonrestful sleep, leading to excessive daytime sleepiness and tiredness.
- Sleepiness and tiredness are not the same but can occur together.
- Sleep apnea, if it is bad enough, can give rise to other medical problems, especially high blood pressure, heart disease, and strokes.
- Other conditions, including diabetes mellitus, acid reflux, hypothyroidism, and gout have been linked to sleep apnea in one way or another.
- Sleep apnea should be treated for two major reasons: to get more restful sleep and to prevent or reduce the risk of other medical conditions.
- Treating sleep apnea often helps not only the person who has it but also the sleep partner.

Chapter 5

Sleep Studies—Taking Out the Mystery

As we saw in the last chapter, sleep apnea is suspected for various reasons and in different situations. Can you decide whether sleep apnea is present and judge the severity just by the symptoms?

Not very well, unfortunately. Although the trend is to have more symptoms (sleepiness, fatigue, etc.) with more severity, the correlation is very rough. It is not unusual for someone with mild sleep apnea to have severe symptoms and for someone with severe sleep apnea to have practically no symptoms. This is probably one of the reasons why a lot of people with sleep apnea never get tested.

We don't fully understand the reasons for this discrepancy between symptoms and severity. One reason may be that people are amazingly variable in their ability to adapt to the effects of apnea: some can cope better than others. Another reason is that symptoms of sleep apnea are also seen with other conditions such as not getting enough sleep. It is sometimes difficult to tell one from the other. Yet another reason is that feeling sleepy or tired is very subjective, and people may maximize or minimize what they feel.

Once the possibility of sleep apnea has been raised for whatever reason, the next step is usually a sleep study, also called a *polysomnogram* or PSG. This is a test performed in a sleep laboratory, a special facility designed to investigate sleep disorders.

The subject sleeps overnight in the sleep laboratory. Data is recorded during sleep by means of small metal probes (electrodes) taped, glued, or fixed with gauze to the scalp and various other parts of the skin. The electrodes are used to record signals to monitor the stages of sleep, snoring, body movements, muscle activity, electrical activity of the heart (EKG), and other processes as required. Special devices record the flow of air as the person breathes in and out. Blood oxygen level is monitored by a special device clipped to a finger or earlobe. Some facilities monitor carbon dioxide, which is produced by the body, in the air that is breathed out. No needles are required. Video monitoring of the sleeping process is also possible.

The different stages of sleep are usually recorded during a sleep study. This helps to interpret the significance of any sleep apnea that may be present. For example, sleep apnea is usually worse in so-called rapid eye movement (REM) sleep, also called "dream sleep." If this stage of sleep is absent or reduced, the severity of sleep apnea can be underestimated. Different positions of sleep are also recorded: sleeping on the back (supine), side sleep, sleeping on the stomach (prone), and sleeping upright. Sleep apnea is often worse during supine sleep—more on this later.

It is important to point out that sleep studies are designed to record data that can be picked up as signals, but not to identify subjective experiences. In other words, it is possible to detect and record sleep stages, pauses in breathing, effort of breathing, heart rhythm, blood oxygen level, and so on. On the other hand, emotion, pain, discomfort, or what the person is dreaming cannot be detected.

Figure 4 shows a diagram of some of the data commonly recorded during a sleep study.

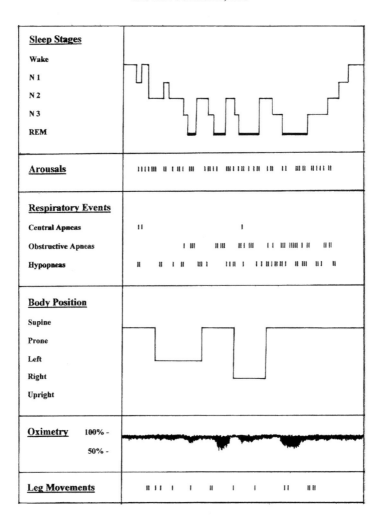

Figure 4. Simplified diagram of data summary from a sleep study

Sleep studies can be tailored for different sleep-related conditions, although in practice, most studies are done for sleep apnea, either to diagnose it or to try treatment for it. A sleep study done to look for sleep apnea (or, less commonly, for another condition) is called a *diagnostic sleep study*. It is important to supply the sleep facility with as much relevant background information as possible to ensure that the test is done for the right reason and with the right equipment.

Modern computer technology has replaced paper recording, but collecting the data is still a very labor-intensive task. After an overnight sleep study, a specially trained technician has to manually examine the data from the entire night *thirty seconds at a time*. For each thirty-second period (known as an "epoch"), the sleep stages, pauses in breathing, oxygen level, etc., have to be noted. This process is called "scoring." The scored study is then interpreted by a physician or other professional trained to read sleep studies. The whole process takes time to do properly, which is why it can be days or even weeks before the final report is ready.

If you are having a sleep study for the first time, it can be quite a daunting prospect, but a little information about the process can allay the anxiety. This chapter should provide answers to some of the questions and concerns about sleep studies. Many sleep laboratories also provide advance information about what a sleep study involves and what one can expect during the night of the study.

Firstly, sleep studies are not done to see how well you sleep in your own home. This would be very difficult because although sleep facilities try to make the sleeping area resemble a normal bedroom, it usually does not feel like home. Sleeping in a strange bed in an unfamiliar room, with electrodes on and being monitored, it is almost expected that you will not sleep as well in the sleep laboratory as you do at home. This can be taken into account when the study is being interpreted, so don't worry about how you will sleep.

Ideal sleep is not required during a sleep study to get a result; as long as sufficient sleep is recorded in various stages, some meaningful information should be available. The process is not perfect, but at present, a sleep study in a sleep laboratory is the best tool we have to gauge the presence and severity of sleep apnea.

Sleep technicians at the sleep facility are trained to conduct the study and record the data. Sometimes they may ask you to sleep in certain positions, even if this is not how you usually sleep—this is because they may require information in that position. Remember that they probably have only one night to collect information and have to make the most of it.

To understand what a sleep study report means, we need to get a little technical and define a few medical terms. *Apnea* means a complete pause in breathing for at least ten seconds. *Hypopnea* refers to shallow breathing, again for at least ten seconds. Hypopneas occur when the air passage is only partially blocked, letting some air pass through. Many apneas and hypopneas are more than ten seconds long, sometimes running into minutes!

Sleep studies are designed to detect apneas as well as hypopneas, both of which are part of what we call sleep apnea. A more accurate name is "sleep apnea-hypopnea syndrome," or SAHS; and when referring to OSA, it is more accurate to call it "obstructive sleep apnea-hypopnea syndrome," or OSAHS. However, to keep things simple, we will use the term "sleep apnea" or simply, "apnea," in this book for OSA. Central sleep apnea (CSA) will only be mentioned as and when required.

The number of apneas and hypopneas during a sleep study are divided by the total number of hours of sleep to give the average number of apneas and hypopneas per hour. This number is called the *apnea-hypopnea index* or AHI, a term commonly seen on a sleep study report. The AHI gives an indication of the severity of the sleep apnea.

An AHI of less than 5 (i.e., less 5 apneas or hypopneas per hour) is considered normal in adults because some pauses in breathing are actually expected in a normal healthy person. An AHI of 5-15 represents mild apnea; 15-30, moderate apnea; and more than 30, severe apnea. An AHI of 30 indicates that the person has thirty interruptions in breathing (apneas plus hypopneas) per hour, which is once every two minutes. In fact, the AHI can be 100 or even higher in extreme cases! Ideally, people with sleep apnea should be aware of their own AHI.

Despite its usefulness, the AHI has some drawbacks and may not always give a true picture of the severity of the apnea. Firstly, the less sleep one gets during a sleep study, the less reliable the AHI becomes, because the sampling time of sleep is short. Secondly, the AHI tells us nothing about other factors that can make sleep apnea mild or severe, such as how low the oxygen level drops. For example, there may not be many apneas or hypopneas, i.e., the AHI may be low, but the oxygen level may drop very low when the person stops breathing. In that case, the low oxygen level gives a more accurate picture of severity and not the AHI. Unfortunately, there is no single number that takes into account all the factors that can affect severity. The AHI is commonly used to indicate the severity of the apnea, but one should look at other factors such as the drop in oxygen level to assess the actual severity.

Another term commonly used in sleep studies is *arousal*. This means a change in the type of brain waves, lasting less than fifteen seconds, often indicating a change from deeper to shallower sleep. Arousals are not the same as awakenings, which mean actual waking up from sleep. A person with sleep apnea has many arousals due to the repeated struggles to breathe. These are called respiratory effort related arousals, or RERAs, and they usually outnumber actual awakenings.

The common idea that a person "wakes up" many times due to sleep apnea refers to RERAs more than to actual awakenings. RERAs can be considered partial awakenings, which do not result in complete alertness. They last only seconds, and people generally have no recollection of them. This is why people with sleep apnea are usually not aware of how many times their sleep is disturbed at night.

Some sleep facilities report a number called respiratory disturbance index or RDI, which includes not only apneas and hypopneas but also RERAs, which indicate sleep disturbance due to breathing problems but do not qualify as apneas or hypopneas. The RDI gives information similar to that obtained from the AHI. Some people use the terms AHI and RDI interchangeably, but strictly speaking, they are not the same. Again, to keep things simple, we will use only the term AHI in this book.

Can you be checked for sleep apnea at home without having a sleep study at a sleep facility? Yes and no. Studies with limited capabilities have been developed to check for sleep apnea at home, but they do not provide all the data that an in-laboratory study can provide. Home studies also lack the benefit of having a trained sleep technician available to troubleshoot if required.

Home studies can give some idea of the likelihood of sleep apnea and can help to decide who should go for a sleep study in a sleep laboratory. Currently, a sleep study in a sleep laboratory is the "gold standard" for diagnosing and assessing sleep apnea. However, technology for home sleep studies is evolving and improving, and we may see more accurate and reliable home sleep studies in the future.

Once a diagnosis of sleep apnea is established, a second sleep study can be done to test the effect of treatment. Usually, this is done to try a type of treatment called *continuous positive airway pressure,* or CPAP. Basically, this involves using a small air pump to blow air at a low pressure into the nose through a mask while the person is sleeping. The technique is described in more detail in chapter 7.

A sleep study done to test the effect of CPAP is called a *CPAP titration study*. The subject is hooked up in the same way as for a diagnostic study, but this time CPAP is started, usually at a low pressure. During the night, the air pressure is gradually adjusted to a level where it controls the sleep apnea (Figure 5). The best pressure level is different for each individual and depends on the severity of the apnea, the person's weight, the structure and floppiness of the upper air passage, and other factors. The titration study also gives the person a chance to see what CPAP feels like so that getting used to it is easier later on.

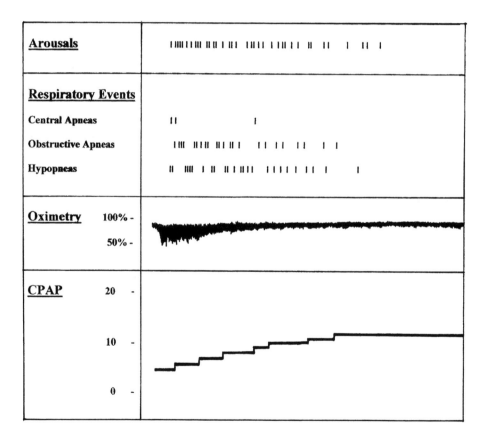

Figure 5. Simplified diagram of CPAP titration, showing
improvement in arousals, respiratory events (apneas and hypopneas),
and oxygen saturation with increasing levels of CPAP

Sleep studies can also be done to assess the effect of other types of treatment for sleep apnea. A person can have a sleep study while using an oral appliance to see if it is working or not. Sleep studies can also be done after surgery to see how effective it has been. The types of treatments available are discussed in more detail in chapter 7.

A simple test called *overnight pulse oximetry* is worth mentioning here. This test involves recording the oxygen level in the blood during the night without the need to draw blood. Using a probe fixed to a finger or earlobe, the equipment basically records the blood oxygen level (or oxygen saturation as it is called) throughout the night. In this way, it is possible to tell whether the oxygen level is dropping significantly at night, one of the features of sleep apnea.

A normal overnight pulse oximetry result does not completely rule out sleep apnea since the pauses in breathing may not be long enough to drop the oxygen level, even though they may occur often enough to disturb sleep. Also, low oxygen levels can occur with other conditions besides sleep apnea, such as certain lung and heart problems. Low oxygen levels on an overnight pulse oximetry test may require more testing for lung or heart conditions and may sometimes require a sleep study to look for sleep apnea.

Overnight pulse oximetry can also be used to check if treatment is effective in someone who has already been found to have sleep apnea, though it is not as reliable as a sleep study.

At a Glance:

- Symptoms are not a reliable way to gauge the presence and severity of sleep apnea; for this, sleep studies are required.
- Sleep studies are done in specially equipped facilities or sleep laboratories.
- The most common reason for doing sleep studies is to look for sleep apnea or to try treatment for it.
- Information obtained on a sleep study can also distinguish OSA (the common type) from CSA (the uncommon type).
- The severity of sleep apnea is usually based on a number called the apnea-hypopnea index or AHI. This is the number of times a person stops breathing (apneas) or comes close to stopping breathing (hypopneas) in one hour.
- Some tests for sleep apnea can be done at home, but they cannot provide as much information as a sleep study in a sleep laboratory. However, better home sleep studies may become available in future.
- Overnight pulse oximetry is a test that measures the oxygen level in the blood at night without the need to draw blood. This test can be used to screen people for sleep apnea, though it cannot confirm the diagnosis.

Chapter 6

Lifestyle Measures to Treat Sleep Apnea

Lifestyle measures are generally underappreciated for the benefits they provide, particularly in today's health care environment in North America, which emphasizes expensive devices and procedures at the expense of more straightforward and commonsense methods.

Weight Loss

Top on the list of lifestyle measures is weight loss. We are rapidly turning, or have turned, into an obese society. Unless we do something about obesity in the general population, sleep apnea will likely become more common in the future. Sleep apnea is more common in overweight and obese people, one reason being the fatty tissue around the neck and throat makes it much easier for the air passage to close off during sleep. A neck circumference of 17 inches or more in men and 16 inches or more in women increases the risk of sleep apnea.

One of the simplest measures of obesity is *waist circumference*. A value of more than 40 inches for men and 34 inches for women is a rough indication of central obesity, i.e., excess weight around the middle of the body. A more accurate classification of adults into normal, overweight, and obese groups is based on the *body mass index* or BMI. This is calculated from the height and weight of an individual (weight in kilograms/square of height in metres = BMI). Usually, a BMI of 20 to 25 is considered the normal range, 25 to 30 represents the overweight range, and more than 30 indicates obesity. The greater the BMI, the greater the possibility of sleep apnea and the more severe it is likely to be.

Weight is a balance between the input and output of energy (calories). When the input is consistently greater than the output, the result is weight gain. In the setting of sleep apnea, gaining weight can set off a vicious cycle of worsening of apnea, which results in daytime sleepiness and fatigue, leading to reduced exercise, which in turn causes more weight gain (Figure 6). This is one of the reasons why people with sleep apnea find it so hard to lose weight, but the cycle has to be broken somewhere if the problem is to be treated.

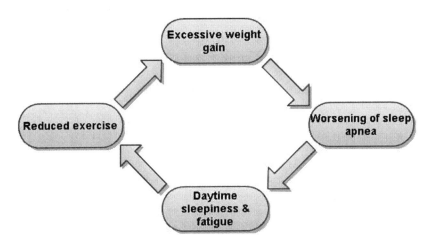

Figure 6. The weight-sleep apnea cycle

On the positive side, it is possible to use the weight-sleep apnea cycle to one's advantage. If one manages to lose some weight, the severity of the sleep apnea can be reduced, making a person less sleepy and lethargic, which in turn makes it easier to become more active and burn off more energy, resulting in more weight loss. In some cases, if the apnea is mild, weight loss may be the only treatment required. According to one source, a 10 percent reduction in weight can result in a 26 percent improvement in sleep apnea.

The problem with weight loss is that one not only needs to lose enough weight but also needs to keep it off. This calls for a lot of self-discipline and perseverance. Any weight loss program can work for sleep apnea as long as one can actually lose weight and keep it off. The actual method is an individual decision—there is no single weight loss program for sleep apnea.

Motivation is crucial to the success of any weight loss program. One way to keep motivated is to keep the benefits in mind—weight loss helps not only sleep apnea but also high blood pressure, heart disease, diabetes, and the risk of certain cancers; it even delays or prevents osteoarthritis of the knees and other weight-bearing joints. As well, losing weight improves mobility and promotes a sense of well-being and accomplishment. In other words, hard though it may be, successful weight loss has many potential benefits.

Weight loss has generally been underemphasized as a treatment option even by health care professionals; sometimes the most obvious solution is also the most neglected one. Few health-related actions have as many benefits as losing weight. Along with smoking cessation, weight loss ranks right up there as one of the most useful measures to improve overall health.

How much weight should one lose? Ideally, the goal should be to achieve an optimal BMI, but even losing less weight is useful if a person is overweight or obese. In my practice, I have found it useful to advise people to lose 10 percent of their current weight as an initial goal, even though some will need to lose more weight later on. This gives them a target to aim for without the need to do calculations or remember any complicated formula.

Weight loss has become a multibillion dollar industry. Despite all the hype about certain weight loss diets, exercises, formulas, supplements, and even pills, the basic principle is simple: weight loss will only occur when the calories used up exceed the calories gained ("burn more than you earn"). Animals, including humans, get their energy from what they eat. There is no "magic formula" for weight loss—most reliable authorities recommend a combination of diet control and exercise. It is important not to fall for fad diets or programs that make claims that one can lose weight despite consuming unlimited quantities of food: this is just not scientifically possible.

Certain medical conditions limit the ability to exercise, making weight loss difficult to achieve. Even then, there are ways to lose weight; it is the total energy expended that has to be more than the total energy taken in. For example, with weakness of the lower limbs or inability to walk, it is possible to do upper body exercises. Water exercises can help people with joint and weight-bearing problems by taking some of the load off weight-bearing joints.

Smoking Cessation

Smokers usually have a lot of congestion and swelling in the nose and upper air passage, which reduces the calibre of the airway. Stopping smoking reduces this problem and makes it less likely to block off during sleep, thus improving sleep apnea. Stopping smoking also has other better-known benefits on the lungs, heart, and brain: much less risk of COPD, less risk of heart problems and strokes, and reduced risk of many types of cancer, to name just a few.

Some smokers gain weight after they quit smoking, mainly because the taste buds recover, appetite improves, and they tend to eat more. This weight gain is usually small and should not be a reason not to quit smoking. The slight weight gain can be reversed with proper motivation, but damage to the lungs and heart from smoking is mostly permanent. Overweight smokers need to quit smoking *and* lose weight, but if one has to choose between stopping smoking and losing weight, the sensible thing to do is to quit smoking first and try to lose weight afterwards.

Avoiding Sleeping Pills

Sleeping pills (also known as sedatives or hypnotics) are *not* part of the treatment of sleep apnea, even though they may be helpful for some other sleep disorders such as insomnia. Sleeping pills tend to make the upper air passage more floppy (and therefore more easily collapsible). They also reduce the "drive" of the brain to breathe, sometimes causing central sleep apnea. For these reasons, sleeping pills can actually worsen sleep apnea by causing a person to stop breathing more often and for longer periods.

Sleeping pills are best avoided when sleep apnea is present. Unfortunately, some people just can't manage without such medications, either because of chronic insomnia or because they have become dependent on the pills after long-time use. In this situation, it is best to talk to your health care provider to discuss other, possibly safer, medications. Sometimes insomnia can be treated without sleeping pills; for example, a nondrug treatment called cognitive behavior therapy (CBT) can be useful.

Avoiding Alcohol Close to Bedtime

Alcohol should be avoided close to bedtime, since it acts pretty much like a sedative. Alcohol taken just before bedtime makes people snore more than usual, and just like other sedatives, it can make sleep apnea worse. Standard advice to anyone with sleep apnea is to avoid alcohol within three to five hours of bedtime to give it time to wash out of the system. Alcohol also causes repeated arousals later in the night, which is another reason to avoid it just before going to sleep.

Avoiding Supine Sleep

Sometimes sleep apnea is present only (or mainly) when the person is asleep on his or her back. In this situation, which is also called *positional apnea*, avoiding sleeping on the back can be effective. Different methods of doing this have been devised, from sewing a tennis ball to the back of the shirt, to using a body pillow, to more complex products available commercially (e.g. "snore balls")—all of which are designed to make sleeping on the back uncomfortable. The problem is you cannot always be sure that the apnea is really positional with information that usually comes from a single sleep study. If there is a doubt, it is probably safer to assume that the apnea is not positional.

In summary, there are many lifestyle measures that can be used to treat sleep apnea. These can be put into practice by anyone who is sufficiently motivated. Depending upon the severity of sleep apnea, they may be all that is required for treatment. Sometimes more than one method is required; for example, one can try losing weight as well as sleeping on one's side.

Even if lifestyle measures do not completely control sleep apnea, they are a useful addition to other methods, which are described in the next chapter.

At a Glance:

- There are many lifestyle measures that can be used to treat sleep apnea. These can be effective by themselves or in combination with other medical treatments.
- Weight loss is recommended for anyone who is overweight or obese, not just for sleep apnea, but because it has other health-related benefits.
- Stopping smoking can reduce sleep apnea by reducing the congestion in the nose and throat.
- Sleeping pills are sedatives and can make sleep apnea worse, even though they may help people with insomnia. They are best avoided or used in the lowest possible dose.
- Alcohol acts as a sedative and also makes sleep apnea worse if taken too close to bedtime. Alcohol also disrupts sleep later in the night.
- Avoiding sleeping on the back is one way to treat positional apnea, which refers to sleep apnea that is present only (or mainly) when the person is sleeping on his or her back.

Chapter 7

CPAP and Other Treatment Methods

Besides the measures mentioned in the previous chapter, sleep apnea can be treated in various other ways, some of which are better known than others.

The best treatment available for sleep apnea (and probably the best known) is *continuous positive airway pressure,* or CPAP, which deserves to be described in some detail. CPAP was first developed in Australia in the early 1980s. A small bedside unit, which is actually an air pump, blows air gently through a mask or other similar device into the nose to create a slight positive air pressure in the floppy rubber-tube-like part of the air passage while the person sleeps. The air pressure acts as an "air splint" to keep the passage open, removes the obstruction, and eliminates the cause of snoring and sleep apnea (Figure 7).

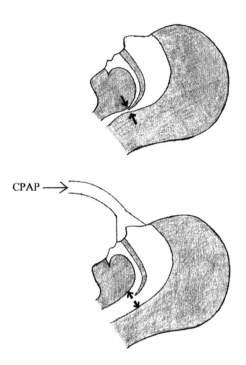

Figure 7. Upper air passage obstruction relieved with CPAP
[Adapted from: *Questions and Answers in Sleep Apnea (An Internist's Perspective)*
by Gautam Soparkar, Xlibris, 2009]

Typical CPAP levels range between four and twenty centimeters of water pressure and can be adjusted to keep the upper air passage open to overcome the obstruction without causing discomfort. Most cases of sleep apnea are controlled at pressures of eight to twelve centimeters of water. The correct pressure is usually found by doing a CPAP titration study (described in chapter 5).

CPAP requires no drugs and no operations. It deals directly with the problem that causes sleep apnea, i.e., the obstruction of the air passage. Contrary to what some people believe, there is no need for tanks of oxygen (although if oxygen is required for other reasons, it can also be supplied through the mask).

Although it may sound uncomfortable to anyone who has not used it, CPAP has really revolutionized the treatment of sleep apnea since it was first introduced in the early 1980s. Over the years, the units have become more compact, more efficient, and even less expensive. The newer models are very quiet and relatively nonintrusive, and there is a wide choice of different types with a variety of features designed to make them comfortable and convenient to use.

CPAP masks have also improved over the years. There are many types, ranging from typical nasal masks that fit only over the nose, to masks that go over the nose and the mouth (suitable for mouth breathers). There are even smaller devices called nasal pillows, which fit snugly in the nostrils, for people who feel claustrophobic with a regular mask.

Mask fitting is an art. Sometimes the first mask is the right fit; at other times, it takes a little patience and effort to find the right fit. The benefits of a well-fitted mask providing just the right pressure are tremendous. For many people, especially those with severe sleep apnea, CPAP is a lifesaver, literally and figuratively, by providing much-needed restful sleep and reducing the risk of high blood pressure and other medical problems.

Modern CPAP units have become more sophisticated in their function, and different modifications have been developed. One such modification is the auto-CPAP unit, which basically self-adjusts the pressure, depending upon what is required in different positions and from night to night. This device is sometimes used to try CPAP at different levels at home, i.e., instead of a CPAP titration study in a sleep laboratory. At other times, auto-CPAP is used for the treatment itself.

One variation of CPAP includes *bilevel positive airway pressure* (BiPAP) where two different pressure levels are used: a higher pressure while breathing in and a lower pressure while breathing out. *Adaptive servo-ventilation* (ASV) is a new variation in which the unit itself monitors the breathing and provides different patterns of pressure according to what is required. These variations may be required in special situations, but for the majority of people with sleep apnea, simple CPAP without any modifications is sufficient. Figure 8 shows a typical CPAP setup with the mask, headgear, hose, and CPAP unit.

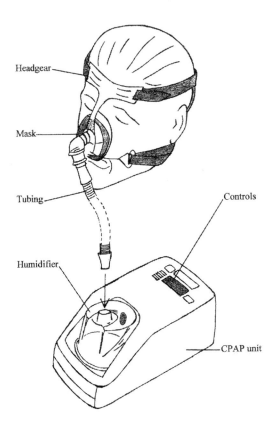

Figure 8. Typical CPAP setup
[Adapted from: *Questions and Answers in Sleep Apnea (An Internist's Perspective)*
by Gautam Soparkar, Xlibris, 2009]

CPAP is almost always effective for sleep apnea, specifically OSA, provided it is used correctly. When it does not work, it is usually because the person cannot or will not use it. Sleep apnea of any severity can be treated with CPAP. For mild to moderate apnea, other options are available (see below), but these are not very effective for severe apnea, for which CPAP is the treatment of choice.

Oral appliances are another way to treat sleep apnea. These are usually provided by dentists or denturists with special expertise in this field. There are two main kinds: those that move the jaw forward and those that adjust the position of the tongue. Both types help reduce snoring and sleep apnea by increasing the space at the back of the throat. Oral appliances are suitable for snoring (without apnea) and for mild to moderate sleep apnea. By themselves, they do not work well for severe apnea, as mentioned above. Jaw pain and tooth discomfort are some of the problems sometimes encountered with these devices.

Surgery is yet another option for the treatment of sleep apnea. There are different types of operations, the most common one being *uvulopalatopharyngoplasty* or UPPP. In this type of surgery, the uvula and part of the soft palate (the flap that hangs down in the throat) are trimmed. This type of operation helps snoring more often than sleep apnea. As with oral appliances, it does not work well for severe cases but can work for mild to moderate apnea and that too in selected individuals.

Some potential drawbacks of such operations include the risk of anesthesia, pain after the surgery (when the anesthetic wears off), and change in the voice. Difficulty with swallowing may occur—usually this is short-lived but can occasionally persist. Consultation with an ear, nose, and throat (ENT) specialist is recommended when such surgery is considered.

If the tonsils or adenoids are enlarged, these can be removed to open up the breathing passage. Big tonsils or adenoids are the most common cause of sleep apnea in children in whom surgery can sometimes completely cure the apnea. In adults, it is rare to find tonsils or adenoids big enough to cause apnea.

An operation to correct a deviated nasal septum (the thin wall that separates the two nasal passages) can improve snoring or mild apnea. This can also help a person adapt better to CPAP by eliminating nasal blockage. Sometimes the back of the tongue can be trimmed if it is too large. Rarely, sleep apnea is due to some anatomical abnormality of the air passage, jaw, or mouth; an operation may be required to correct the problem.

Mild apnea can often be treated with lifestyle measures alone, unless the person has a lot of symptoms or other medical conditions, in which case additional treatment may be required. CPAP, oral appliances and surgery are all reasonable options for mild to moderate apnea, depending upon the circumstances. Severe apnea generally requires CPAP as the first-choice treatment, with other options to be considered only if this is not possible.

Before CPAP became available, the only effective treatment for severe sleep apnea was a *tracheostomy*. This is basically an opening in the windpipe made surgically through the front of the lower neck, through which a tube is placed. During the day, the opening can be covered, and the person can breathe normally through the nose. At night, the opening is uncovered and the person breathes through it, bypassing the obstruction in the upper airway and eliminating sleep apnea. Tracheostomy is still performed for very severe and life-threatening apnea but is rarely required, now that CPAP is available.

Weight loss surgery is a form of operation performed for extremely obese people who cannot lose weight by other methods. It is also known as *bariatric surgery*, or gastric bypass surgery, although the stomach is not actually bypassed in many cases. Variations of such surgery include procedures like laparoscopic banding, which is done through a tiny opening instead of requiring a big incision. Usually, such surgery is done when there is severe obesity (defined as a BMI of more than 40), and other weight loss methods have failed. People typically lose a lot of weight after such surgery, and this type of treatment has been quite successful (in properly selected candidates) for sleep apnea, even though it may or may not eliminate it completely.

Sometimes combining different treatments works better than one treatment alone. For example, people with nasal blockage often have trouble tolerating CPAP through a nasal mask. Nasal blockage can also make an oral appliance feel suffocating. Correcting the blockage with medications or surgery can make it easier to use CPAP or oral appliances.

Medications have been tried for sleep apnea but with limited success. Generally, medications to eliminate the obstruction in OSA are not very useful, but treatment of nasal obstruction with anti-inflammatory sprays or decongestants can reduce snoring and sometimes help mild sleep apnea by reducing the swelling of the lining and increasing the patency of the nose.

Occasionally, drugs that encourage the drive to breathe (so-called respiratory stimulants) are used along with other treatments like CPAP. By themselves, such medications are not very effective for OSA because the problem is mainly a mechanical one (obstruction of the upper air passage). Respiratory stimulants are more useful in CSA, where obstruction is not the problem (see below).

Some medications keep people awake and alert. One example is a drug called *modafinil*. This drug is often used in other sleep disorders like narcolepsy but can sometimes be taken when troublesome sleepiness persists even after sleep apnea has been treated adequately with CPAP or other methods. However, not all experts agree with this type of treatment because the medication only treats the sleepiness, not the apnea itself.

CSA is much less common than OSA but is more difficult to treat. For the most part, treatment of central sleep apnea means treating the illness that caused it, which can be heart failure or certain brain disorders. Drugs that suppress brain activity, such as sleeping pills and narcotics, can cause or worsen CSA and should be avoided if possible. CPAP can be used for CSA but may or may not work. Oxygen is sometimes useful.

Certain medications can be useful to get the breathing centres in the brain to send the right signals to the lungs. A drug called *acetazolamide* (also used to treat mountain sickness) has shown some promise in the treatment of central sleep apnea. It is usually taken in a small dose at bedtime and can help central sleep apnea by providing sufficient stimulation to the brain to eliminate or reduce the pauses in breathing.

Often, sleep apnea is not the only issue but adds to problems caused by insufficient sleep or other causes of non-restful sleep, such as certain medical illnesses or chronic pain. All these problems result in feeling excessively sleepy or tired during the day. This may be one of the reasons why treatment of sleep apnea is sometimes not successful or only partly successful. This is not a true failure—it is just that other causes of nonrestful sleep have not been resolved. In order to get truly restful sleep, the other problems need to be addressed.

The above-mentioned methods of treatment are only guidelines: the actual choice of treatment should be made only after discussion with a qualified healthcare professional, taking into account the type and severity of the apnea, symptoms, presence or absence of other medical conditions, occupation, and personal preferences. Any of these factors can change the final treatment plan.

The bottom line is that there are many ways to treat sleep apnea. One size does not fit all: treatment should be individualized as much as possible. Some treatments are more effective than others, but it is a common mistake to assume that there is only one type of treatment available for sleep apnea.

At a Glance:

- For OSA (the most common type), the best treatment is CPAP. This technique can be used for mild, moderate or severe apnea but is most necessary when the apnea is severe. Typically, people with sleep apnea get more restful sleep and feel more refreshed and alert with CPAP.
- Oral appliances and surgery are reasonable options if the sleep apnea is mild to moderate in severity. Dental appliances and commonly performed operations are unlikely to provide complete relief from severe apnea unless combined with other methods.
- Tracheostomy is a type of surgery that is very effective for OSA but is now used only in severe, life-threatening situations.
- CSA is more difficult to treat and often involves treating the cause. Sometimes CPAP works for this condition. At other times, medications or oxygen may be useful.
- There are many ways to treat sleep apnea. Treatment should be individualized for each person.

Chapter 8

Sleep Apnea and Special Situations

Upper Airway Resistance Syndrome

A special condition called upper airway resistance syndrome, or UARS, needs to be mentioned here. This is a type of sleep apnea, but actual apneas or hypopneas are either missing or very few in number. To understand this, let us go back to the rubber tube concept of the upper air passage.

Suppose the tube becomes narrow repeatedly during sleep, not enough to produce apneas or hypopneas, but sufficient to disturb sleep by causing repeated arousals. Technically, these arousals are so-called respiratory effort related arousals or RERAs (see chapter 5). They can prevent the person from getting restful sleep, just like in regular sleep apnea, but without actual apneas or hypopneas. What will show up on the sleep study is increased number of arousals, usually with snoring, but hardly any apneas or hypopneas. This is called upper airway resistance syndrome, or UARS. It is basically a kind of sleep apnea, but the disturbed sleep is because of the arousals without actual interruptions in breathing. UARS can have the same effect on sleep quality and produce the same symptoms as regular sleep apnea.

UARS should be suspected when a sleep study shows many arousals but few, if any, apneas or hypopneas. However, most sleep facilities cannot confirm UARS without special equipment, which is generally available only in specialized laboratories designed for research. Since there are many other reasons for having arousals, the diagnosis of UARS is usually confirmed by trying some treatment, usually CPAP. Improvement in sleep quality with treatment then indicates that UARS is present.

Once UARS is detected, it is treated in much the same way as regular sleep apnea.

Sleep Apnea in Children

Children can also have sleep apnea. Unlike in adults, where obesity is one of the biggest risk factors, the most common cause of snoring and sleep apnea in children is big tonsils or adenoids. However, excess weight can add to the problem, and sleep apnea may become more common in children in the future because of the growing epidemic of childhood obesity.

Children may not show the classic symptoms of sleepiness and tiredness—sometimes they are actually overactive. This can sometimes result in a wrong diagnosis; for example, children may be labeled as having attention deficit hyperactivity disorder (ADHD) or some other condition. At other times, they may not show any obvious symptoms, but their performance at school might suffer.

A detailed discussion of sleep apnea in children is beyond the scope of this book, but it is important to emphasize that children can also have sleep apnea, and the symptoms are often quite different from those seen in adults.

Pickwickian Syndrome

The term "Pickwickian syndrome" comes from Charles Dickens's description of the obese boy in his book *The Pickwick Papers*. The medical name of this condition is *obesity hypoventilation syndrome* (OHS). In this condition, not only is there sleep apnea but also so much obesity that it actually interferes with the working of the muscles of breathing, resulting in shallow breaths. People with this condition have trouble moving air in and out of the lungs, not just during sleep, but even when they are awake.

Besides low blood oxygen levels, the carbon dioxide levels in the blood are high, and this produces the typical red face. Usually, the brain is quite sensitive to build-up of carbon dioxide and fights this by increasing the rate and depth of breathing. In the Pickwickian syndrome, this sensitivity is lost, and breathing remains shallow. Extreme sleepiness results from non-restful sleep (because of sleep apnea) and the high carbon dioxide level.

People with the Pickwickian syndrome are at particularly high risk of other medical problems, even more so than those with regular sleep apnea. A particular type of high blood pressure that occurs only in the blood vessels of the lungs, called pulmonary artery hypertension (PAH), is much more common with the Pickwickian syndrome than with regular sleep apnea. This can result in strain on the right side of the heart.

Treatment of this condition is similar to that of regular sleep apnea, with more emphasis on weight loss and CPAP.

Overlap Syndrome

Sleep apnea is very common in the general population, and so is another condition known as chronic obstructive pulmonary disease (COPD), which is usually the result of smoking for many years. It is only to be expected that some people will have both.

The combination of sleep apnea and COPD has been called overlap syndrome and is a particularly risky scenario since both conditions cause the oxygen level to drop. Even if the oxygen level is normal while awake, it can drop precipitously during sleep, particularly in REM sleep, putting the person more at risk than if only one condition was present.

Depending upon how low the blood oxygen drops, people with the overlap syndrome may require oxygen at night along with CPAP. If they are smokers, stopping smoking is important to prevent further worsening of the COPD. They also require appropriate treatment for COPD with inhalers and possibly other medications during the day.

Sleep Apnea in Pregnancy

Pregnant women can get sleep apnea even with the normal weight gain and hormonal changes of pregnancy. Sleep apnea in pregnancy is more common if the woman was overweight before pregnancy. The good news is that if there was no sleep apnea before pregnancy, there is every reason to expect that the apnea will disappear when weight loss occurs after the pregnancy is over.

Some snoring can occur even in otherwise normal pregnancy because of weight gain and nasal congestion, which is due to hormones. Tiredness can be due to the pregnancy itself. This is why sleep apnea is often not suspected in pregnancy. Although there is no need to look for sleep apnea in every pregnant woman, some clues might point that way. Loud snoring, excessive sleepiness or fatigue, or too much weight gain should prompt a discussion about sleep apnea with the health care provider. A sleep study can then be arranged if required.

Sleep apnea during pregnancy is different from other situations because treatment is required not only for the mother but also because low oxygen levels can be risky for the baby. Another difference is that losing weight is not generally recommended in pregnancy unless the weight gain is dangerously excessive. Weight loss should never be undertaken in pregnancy except under close medical supervision. If the apnea is bad enough, the mother may require treatment with CPAP during the pregnancy. After delivery, many (if not most) mothers can stop the treatment once the weight comes off.

Sleep Apnea and Depression

Sleep apnea has been reported to be a cause of depression. Whether this is real depression or just looks like depression is a matter of opinion. What is clear is that many people with sleep apnea feel low and sad, showing the same symptoms as people who are depressed. To some extent, this may be because of the disruption of sleep itself, which can occur not only with sleep apnea but with many other sleep disorders. Sleep apnea can cause problems at work or in relationships, which can, in turn, lead to depression. Whatever the reason for the depression-like symptoms with sleep apnea, treatment of the apnea can often improve the symptoms, if not eliminate them completely.

Sleep apnea should be considered in anybody who seems to be depressed and is also overweight and snores. A sleep study should be considered in these circumstances—it might bring to light sleep apnea, which was previously not recognized. One particular risk of not picking up sleep apnea in this situation is that people may be started on antidepressants, some of which have sleeping pill-like qualities and can actually worsen sleep apnea.

Sleep Apnea and General Anesthesia

A general anesthetic can make sleep apnea worse for much the same reasons as sleeping pills and alcohol: it makes the upper air passage more floppy and more collapsible. Surgeons and anesthesiologists like to know in advance whether or not a person undergoing an operation has sleep apnea so that special precautions can be taken. Usually, the person is required to start treatment, often with CPAP, before the operation.

Many people with sleep apnea are also obese and have narrow upper airways. This makes it more difficult to pass a tube (called an endotracheal tube) in the upper air passage, something that is done routinely for an operation under general anesthesia. If this is the case, it is better to know in advance so that plans for anesthesia can be modified appropriately.

Sleep Apnea in People Going For Weight Loss Surgery (Bariatric Surgery)

People going for weight loss surgery are often required to have a sleep study before the operation. One reason is the risk of worsening apnea with anesthesia (see above).

The second reason is that practically everyone going for such surgery is severely obese (usually with a BMI of 40 or more) and, therefore, at fairly high risk of sleep apnea. A sleep study can show if there is sleep apnea. Depending upon the severity, treatment with CPAP may have to be started before the operation. After surgery and when sufficient weight loss has occurred, the sleep study can be repeated to see if the sleep apnea has improved.

At a Glance:

- Upper airway resistance syndrome (UARS) is a condition where there is repeated narrowing of the upper air passage, causing arousals and disturbance of sleep, but no obvious apneas or hypopneas. Symptoms and treatment are similar to those of regular sleep apnea.
- Sleep apnea can occur in children. The symptoms may be different from those seen in adults. Enlarged tonsils or adenoids are the usual cause of sleep apnea in these cases.
- The term "Pickwickian syndrome" includes sleep apnea with obesity that is severe enough to cause shallow breathing even during the day. People with this condition are at even greater risk of other medical problems than those with regular sleep apnea.
- The overlap syndrome refers to sleep apnea and chronic obstructive pulmonary disease (COPD) occurring in the same individual. Severe drops in oxygen level at night can occur as a result of this combination.
- Pregnancy is a special situation in which treatment of apnea should take into account the needs of the mother and the unborn baby. Weight loss is not part of the usual treatment in pregnancy.
- Sleep apnea can cause depression or at least produce symptoms very similar to depression. Treatment of the apnea can often relieve or cure this "depression." Some antidepressant medications can make sleep apnea worse.
- General anesthesia tends to make sleep apnea worse. Surgeons and anesthesiologists usually like to know in advance about any sleep apnea that may be present so that appropriate precautions can be taken.
- A sleep study is often done before weight loss surgery, firstly because of the concerns with general anesthesia and, secondly, because severe obesity makes sleep apnea more likely. Another sleep study can be done after weight loss occurs to check for improvement.

Chapter 9

Putting It All Together

So where are we today with sleep apnea?

We now know sleep apnea is very common. We are aware that it can disrupt day-to-day life because of sleepiness, fatigue, and other symptoms. We have also recently learned that it plays a role in many other health issues: high blood pressure, heart problems, strokes, diabetes—the list goes on. Many people who see their health care provider for seemingly unrelated problems have sleep apnea, at least to some degree. There is also good and effective treatment available for it.

We now have better technology to diagnose the condition, more options for treatment, and better equipment to make treatment acceptable for more people than ever before. Yet the unfortunate reality is that many people with sleep apnea do not benefit from these advances. There are several reasons for this:

1. Sleep apnea is a relatively new subject: even many health care professionals don't know much about it.
2. Sleep apnea gets less priority compared to other conditions simply because it is considered a "sleep" disorder.
3. Sleep apnea and its consequences are still not well-known among the general public. Most people seriously underestimate the effect of this condition on their level of alertness and their health.
4. There are many misconceptions about the condition.

In my opinion, the main problem is that sleep apnea does not come to mind readily, both for health care providers and patients. It is simply not on the map when someone is being assessed medically. Awareness needs to improve and misconceptions need to be dispelled before sleep apnea can be recognized and treated, much the same as for any other health condition. Teaching in medical and nursing schools needs to incorporate sleep apnea as a major medical problem, rather than some sort of "fringe" condition.

Sleep apnea should be considered a public health issue for two major reasons:

Firstly, sleep apnea is an important (though not the only) cause of daytime sleepiness. Sleepiness is pervasive in our society today, with sleep apnea, other sleep disorders, shift work, long waking hours, and a host of other situations all competing to whittle away at our sleep time and quality. The news is full of accidents, injuries, and deaths due to sleepy people who were just not up to the task at hand, putting their own lives and those of others on the line.

Secondly, as we have seen, sleep apnea is related, directly or indirectly, to so many other health issues that it is impossible to compute the cost in terms of human productivity, lives, and illnesses. All we can say with confidence is that as our population ages and as conditions like obesity becomes more common, there is every reason to believe that sleep apnea will become more and more of a problem, and dealing with it on a population basis will become more necessary.

Until sleep apnea is recognized as a public health issue, it will continue to be underdiagnosed and undertreated. In the words of Dr. William Dement, the father of modern sleep medicine and pioneer researcher in sleep:

> *In recent years, we have learned that pervasive sleep deprivation and undiagnosed sleep disorders are arguably our largest health problem. A single sleep problem, obstructive sleep apnea, is now known to afflict 30 million people. If unrecognized in its advanced stages, this disorder is disabling and eventually lethal. If recognized and treated, even those who are near death's door can be saved and restored to normal health.*

At a Glance:

- Sleep apnea is underrecognized because of inadequate knowledge and misconceptions among health care personnel and the public.
- The risks of untreated sleep apnea are so great in terms of sleepiness and health risks that it should be treated as a public health issue.

Chapter 10

Frequently Asked Questions

Sleep Apnea in General

1. I think I sleep well—so well that I fall asleep as soon as my head hits the pillow. Can I still have sleep apnea?

Yes. Most people with sleep apnea are not aware they have it because they are asleep when it occurs. Falling asleep as soon as your head hits the pillow is actually a sign of excessive sleepiness, of which sleep apnea is one cause.

Sleep apnea is not just about not sleeping well. It means stopping (or coming close to stopping) breathing in your sleep. If you snore loudly and don't feel refreshed when you wake up, are unduly sleepy during the day, have a headache first thing in the morning, or have any of the symptoms linked to sleep apnea in chapter 4, you may have sleep apnea. Additional risk factors are being overweight and having another condition such as high blood pressure, which increase the chances of having sleep apnea even if symptoms are not present.

2. I feel very sleepy and tired during the day. Does that mean I have sleep apnea?

Not necessarily, but you *may* have sleep apnea. Many situations can produce non-restful sleep, such as not sleeping for long enough, an uncomfortable bed, extremes of heat and cold, anxiety, depression, pain, and other health-related issues, to name just a few. Sleep apnea is just one of the conditions which can make you feel sleepy and tired during the day. Clues that your problem may be sleep apnea include being overweight, snoring (especially if it is loud), and someone actually seeing you stop breathing while you sleep. The presence of some medical conditions such as high blood pressure are additional indirect clues that you might have sleep apnea. The best way to find out is by getting a sleep study.

3. What are the common health conditions associated with sleep apnea?

Sleep apnea increases the risk of developing high blood pressure. About half the people with untreated apnea have high blood pressure, and about a third of people with high blood pressure have sleep apnea. High blood pressure by itself can lead to heart problems, strokes, and kidney disease, compounding the health problems.

Sleep apnea by itself increases the chances of having heart problems and strokes. Recent information suggests that the risk of type 2 diabetes and gout is also higher with sleep apnea.

Many of these conditions are more common in overweight people, but if a person also has sleep apnea, the risk is even higher.

4. I am not overweight. Can I still have sleep apnea?

Yes. Sleep apnea is more common and more severe in overweight or obese people, but a person of normal weight can also have sleep apnea, depending upon the structure and floppiness of the upper air passage. Sleep apnea also becomes more common as one gets older, although this is not always the case.

Talk to your health care provider if you have symptoms of sleep apnea or if you have a medical condition that commonly goes along with sleep apnea. You might require a sleep study even if your weight is normal.

5. I have sleep apnea. How do I decide on the best treatment?

The best treatment is one that is tailored for you, taking into account the severity of your apnea, how much it is affecting your life, your occupation, and any other medical conditions you may have. The treatment should be planned in consultation with your healthcare provider, who should have a good idea of your health profile. In general, the milder the sleep apnea and its symptoms, the more options you have for treatment.

Severe apnea usually cannot be treated well with certain methods like oral appliances alone. CPAP is usually the treatment of choice in such cases. Sometimes a combination of methods is required.

6. *Can I die from sleep apnea at night?*

Sleep apnea does occasionally cause sudden death at night, likely due to an abnormal heart rhythm (arrhythmia), which stops the pumping action of the heart. This is more likely to happen if the apnea is severe or if there is already an underlying heart or lung problem.

Contrary to what many people believe, interruption of breathing by itself rarely causes death in people with sleep apnea. Most of the time, the breathing resumes after an episode of apnea, even if it is a long pause. This has to happen over and over again to be called sleep apnea, and the odds of not starting to breathe after an episode of apnea are extremely low.

7. *Apart from medical conditions, what is the other major risk of sleep apnea?*

Sleep apnea can make people sleepy and tired. Sometimes these symptoms are so bad that people are at risk while performing tasks that demand alertness, such as driving and flying aircraft. Sometimes the persons involved may not even know the extent to which sleep apnea is affecting their alertness. For example, people can suffer from "microsleeps" (chapter 4), which are extra-brief episodes of sleepiness that can occur without the person being aware of them. These episodes can be catastrophic if they occur at a time when continuous vigilance is required.

8. *Will my sleep apnea get worse as I get older?*

It is difficult to be sure. Sleep apnea does tend to become more common and worse with age, but it is hard to predict who will get worse and who will not. With age, the muscles holding the air passage open become more lax—this is part of the problem, but there is not much we can do about it. Certain medications can make sleep apnea worse, and people tend to require more medications as they get older because of other unrelated health issues. Weight gain is the other reason sleep apnea gets worse with age.

Your best bet for reducing the risk of sleep apnea is to avoid putting on weight, something which unfortunately happens all too often as we get older.

9. *I had a sleep study because of high blood pressure. I have no symptoms but was found to have severe sleep apnea. Should I still have treatment?*

Yes. Treatment is recommended even if you have no symptoms, especially since you have severe sleep apnea, which increases the risk of worsening of blood pressure or developing other problems such as heart disease and strokes. Treating the apnea properly will reduce your risk of these conditions. The high blood pressure may even be the result of sleep apnea, and it is not uncommon for blood pressure to improve once the apnea is treated. Some people are able to reduce or even come off blood pressure medications if this happens.

CPAP will likely be part of the treatment since your apnea is severe. If you have severe apnea but are not offered CPAP just because you have no symptoms, make it a point to find out why.

10. *I have high blood pressure and have had a heart attack. Should I be checked for sleep apnea?*

It may be a good idea to at least bring it up with your healthcare provider, especially if you have symptoms which suggest sleep apnea or are overweight. Sleep apnea is one of the most under-recognized medical conditions, which is unfortunate because it is also very treatable.

When it is moderate to severe, sleep apnea increases the risk of having high blood pressure, heart problems, and strokes. If you already have any of these conditions, sleep apnea may be at least partly responsible, and treating it may reduce your risk of future health problems.

11. I am going to have surgery under general anesthesia. Should I be concerned about sleep apnea?

People with sleep apnea can stop breathing while they are under a general anesthetic. If you are overweight and have symptoms of sleep apnea such as loud snoring and sleepiness, you might want to mention this to your surgeon or anesthesiologist. You may even be asked these questions during your checkup before the operation.

If your surgeon or anesthesiologist feels you might have sleep apnea, they may order a sleep study before your operation. If you have sleep apnea, it does not necessarily mean you cannot have a general anesthetic, but you may need special arrangements and extra precautions, especially just after surgery.

12. Can I use sleeping pills if I have sleep apnea?

In general, using sleeping pills is not a good idea if you have sleep apnea. Sleeping pills help people fall asleep and stay asleep. Although they can help people who have insomnia, they can actually make sleep apnea worse by making the muscles of the upper air passage more floppy, resulting in more and longer pauses in breathing. This can also happen in people who drink alcohol just before sleeping, which is not a good idea even for people without sleep apnea. Alcohol not only worsens sleep apnea but can also cause interrupted sleep in the later part of the night—a phenomenon called "sleep fragmentation."

Unfortunately, some people with sleep apnea just cannot do without sleeping pills, either because they have bad insomnia or because they have become dependent on the pills. In such a situation, it may be best to use the lowest possible dose. If you have sleep apnea but also have to use sleeping pills, talk to your doctor—you may need a lower dose or a different and safer medication. If you are taking sleeping pills for insomnia, ask about other (non-drug) methods of treating this problem, such as cognitive behavior therapy (CBT).

13. My partner is on treatment for depression, but he/she is also overweight and snores loudly. Should he/she be checked for sleep apnea?

The answer is probably yes, especially if the treatment for depression is not working. Sleep apnea may or may not be the reason for the "depression," but the association of snoring and being overweight should certainly raise a red flag, if nothing else. If sleep apnea is found and treated, the symptoms of "depression" may improve or even resolve completely.

The other reason for checking for sleep apnea in this situation is that some (but not all) antidepressant medications also act as sleeping pills and can make sleep apnea worse.

14. Is "sleep-disordered breathing" the same as "sleep apnea"?

Many people use the term "sleep-disordered breathing" and "sleep apnea" to mean the same thing. In fact, sleep apnea is a type of sleep-disordered breathing, which includes other conditions that interfere with breathing during sleep. These include asthma, chronic obstructive pulmonary disease (COPD), and some other less common breathing disorders.

Sometimes more than one condition is present; for example, the same person can have sleep apnea and COPD, a condition called "overlap syndrome." In this situation, the oxygen level in the blood can drop much lower at night than with either condition alone.

Sleep Studies

15. What is a diagnostic sleep study, and what information can it provide?

This is a test done in a sleep laboratory to study sleep. The subject usually sleeps overnight in the sleep laboratory. Data is recorded by means of many electrodes attached to various parts of the body. Information about sleep stages, breathing patterns, oxygen level, heart rhythm, etc., is recorded and later analyzed to produce a report.

The vast majority of diagnostic sleep studies are done to look for sleep apnea and to assess its severity. Sleep studies can detect interruptions in breathing, which can be either total (apneas) or partial (hypopneas). The apnea-hypopnea index (the number of apneas and/or hypopneas per hour), or AHI, gives an idea of the severity of sleep apnea. Other information such as the oxygen level also helps to determine the severity.

16. How can you differentiate the two main types of sleep apnea on a sleep study?

Obstructive sleep apnea (OSA) would show up as no breathing (apnea) or shallow breathing (hypopnea), with the signals of breathing effort being intact. Central sleep apnea (CSA) would show up as apnea with no signals of breathing effort (chapter 2, figure 1).

When the term "sleep apnea" is used, it generally refers to OSA because it is so much more common; although strictly speaking, one should specify whether it is OSA or CSA.

17. What information can a sleep study not *provide?*

Sleep studies are designed to detect and record data that can be picked up as signals; for example: stages of sleep, heart rhythm, pauses in breathing, blood oxygen level, and so on. Subjective experiences like pain, discomfort, and emotional states cannot be recorded with current technology. Similarly, contents of dreams cannot be picked up (although it is possible to detect the so-called dream stage or REM sleep).

Sleep studies are normally not useful for insomnia, since it is unlikely that any result would help to either make the diagnosis or decide on the treatment.

For all their benefits, sleep studies are time-consuming and cumbersome. Sleep studies should be arranged with a clear idea of what one is looking for, and a request for a sleep study should specify why it is being requested. This is an important point since, unfortunately, many sleep studies are done for no good reason.

18. Why can't I get the results of my sleep study immediately after it is done?

Recording and interpreting a sleep study report is a very labor-intensive process (chapter 5). Data on sleep stages, pauses in breathing, heart rhythm, oxygen level, and other variables is collected during the overnight study. This is not the end of the process but just the beginning. A trained sleep technician has to examine the data from the entire night *thirty seconds at a time*, a process known as "scoring." Although the collection process is electronic, the actual scoring process is *manual* and, therefore, time-consuming. The scored information is then interpreted by a physician or other trained health care professional to produce the final report.

The whole process can take days or even weeks, although sleep laboratories can usually expedite the process if they are made aware of an urgent situation.

> *19. Can I be tested for sleep apnea with a daytime nap instead of having to go through an overnight sleep study?*

Overnight sleep usually includes periods of REM (rapid eye movement) sleep, during which sleep apnea is at its worst. REM sleep typically occurs in cycles, usually beginning one and a half to two hours after falling asleep. Cycles of REM sleep get longer in the second half of the night. Daytime naps are usually too short to pick up REM sleep, and lack of this stage of sleep may result in sleep apnea being underestimated or completely missed. For this reason, an overnight sleep study is the preferred way to test for sleep apnea.

Exceptions can be made for people whose sleep pattern involves sleeping in the day and staying awake at night, e.g., people on night shifts. In such cases, daytime sleep studies can be arranged, but the duration is kept long enough to include at least some REM sleep.

> *20. My sleep study report says I have "positional sleep apnea." What does this mean?*

This means you have sleep apnea only (or mainly) when you sleep on your back. Sometimes the tongue slides back in the throat, blocking the air passage and producing sleep apnea. This is most likely to happen if you are sleeping on your back.

If you have positional apnea, you may be able to get around the problem by avoiding sleeping on your back. This can be done by attaching some object, such as a tennis ball, to the back of your nightshirt or by using a body pillow or similar object to keep yourself on your side.

21. *I am going for weight loss surgery. Do I need a sleep study before the operation?*

Many centers offering weight loss surgery require the patient to have a sleep study before the operation. There are two main reasons for this:

(i) Severe obesity, the reason for the operation, increases the chances of sleep apnea, whether or not symptoms are present.

(ii) Having sleep apnea can cause problems if a general anesthetic is given, because general anesthetics increase the risk of stopping breathing in people who have sleep apnea.

Knowing whether or not a person has sleep apnea helps the surgeon and anesthesiologist prepare better for problems that may arise before, during or after surgery. It is preferable to treat moderate to severe sleep apnea adequately before the operation. The treatment can be reassessed when significant weight loss occurs after having the operation.

22. *I had a sleep study in a sleep laboratory but did not sleep well. Is the study any good?*

Many people don't sleep well in a sleep laboratory because of the unfamiliar atmosphere, having to sleep with electrodes attached, and being monitored. This is entirely expected and can be taken into account when the sleep study is read and reported. Even with less-than-usual sleep time and quality, it is possible to obtain a reasonable result.

A lot of people tend to underestimate the amount of sleep they get (because they are asleep!). If you have a sleep study, you may be surprised at how much sleep was actually recorded. It is rare for someone to get no sleep at all during a full night in a sleep facility.

23. *For several years, I have had a hard time falling asleep, or if I wake up in the night, I have had trouble getting back to sleep. Do I need a sleep study?*

Not necessarily. Sleep studies are done mainly to look for sleep apnea. Your symptoms suggest you might have *chronic insomnia* (difficulty getting to or staying asleep). This is a completely different problem and usually requires a different approach. Insomnia has many causes and is often due to one or more factors such as stress, anxiety, depression, physical discomfort, and pain. None of these can be confirmed on a sleep study. Diagnosis of chronic insomnia involves, among other things, a detailed history of the problem, how it started, and what makes it better or worse. A sleep study is unlikely to be helpful if you have insomnia, except, of course, if you also happen to have sleep apnea (some people may have both).

24. I have been asked to have a CPAP titration study. What is involved?

This is a sleep study designed to try CPAP, usually after the diagnosis of sleep apnea has been made. You will be hooked up just like during a diagnostic sleep study, only this time, you will be using CPAP. During the night, the technician will try different levels of CPAP to find out what pressure works best for you.

The study also gives you a chance to try CPAP in the controlled setting of the laboratory. Later on, if you need CPAP, your healthcare provider will probably use the information from the CPAP titration study to set the correct level for you.

25. What is a CPAP autotitration study?

This is a test done with a CPAP autotitrating unit (one which self-adjusts the CPAP level) to try CPAP and find out the best level. Sometimes it is not practical to do a CPAP titration study in a sleep laboratory, and an autotitration study is used in its place. While nothing can replace a CPAP titration study in a sleep facility, where a technician is available to troubleshoot if required, autotitration has the advantage of being cheaper and more convenient since it is usually carried out at home. It can also be carried out over several nights, which may help the subject get used to CPAP.

With the increasing demand for tests for sleep apnea, home autotitration studies may become more popular in the future, freeing up spots in sleep facilities to diagnose sleep apnea.

26. My doctor wants me to have a "split night" sleep study. What does this mean?

Usually, an initial sleep study is done to detect sleep apnea and assess its severity. This is usually followed by a second sleep study to try CPAP. A "split night" sleep study is both studies combined into one—the first part to detect and assess the severity of sleep apnea and the second part to try CPAP.

The advantage of a split study is the convenience of getting two studies done in one night. The main downside is that sometimes there is just not enough time in one night to get all the necessary information, leading to inconclusive results.

27. I have all the symptoms of sleep apnea, but my sleep study did not show any apnea. How is this possible?

Sleep studies can miss sleep apnea in some situations:

- If there are technical problems with recording the signals.
- If certain stages of sleep are missing during the study. Sleep apnea is more common in deep sleep and so-called REM sleep, when the muscles are most relaxed.
- If sleep is not recorded with the person sleeping on his/her back—this is when sleep apnea is usually at its worst.

If there is a strong suspicion that sleep apnea was missed, the sleep study may have to be repeated.

28. Besides sleep apnea, is there any other reason to do a sleep study?

Less commonly, sleep studies are done to look for periodic limb movement disorder (related to but not the same as restless legs syndrome), nighttime seizures, or a condition called narcolepsy (this requires a nighttime *and* a special daytime study known as an MSLT). Rarely, sleep studies may be done for other conditions. Sleep studies may or may not be helpful for all these conditions, and not all authorities agree on all the reasons for doing sleep studies.

CPAP and Other Treatments

29. What is CPAP and how does it work?

CPAP stands for *continuous positive airway pressure*. The technique involves blowing air at a gentle pressure through a mask fitted over the nose into the upper air passage to keep it open during sleep ("air splint") so that the person with sleep apnea can breathe at night without interruptions. CPAP works for all severities of sleep apnea and is particularly useful for the obstructive kind (OSA). It is most required when the apnea is moderate to severe, because most other methods of treatment don't work very well in that situation.

30. My doctor has recommended a CPAP unit for me, but I don't think I can get used to it. Should I refuse the treatment?

Your doctor probably has a good reason for recommending CPAP. Before you refuse the treatment, consider the following: How severe is your sleep apnea? The more severe it is, the more CPAP is necessary. How bad are your symptoms? The more sleepy and tired you are, the more you will probably benefit from CPAP. Do you have other medical problems like high blood pressure or heart disease? If so, CPAP is more important for you.

Look at it this way: If you wear glasses, you would probably prefer not to use them—but you need them to see properly, and so you persist with them. Eventually you get used to them. Similarly, if CPAP is necessary for you, it only makes sense to persist with it.

31. Is a CPAP unit noisy?

Older CPAP units emitted a "white noise" that disturbed some people. Even this noise was usually less intrusive than snoring. Newer units are much more quiet, and sometimes it is difficult to even tell if they are running or not. In any case, there are ways of getting around the problem of noise, such as putting a piece of foam under the unit or placing the unit farther from the bed and getting a longer length of tubing.

Noise should not be a reason for not being able to use CPAP. Talk to your CPAP supplier if this is an issue.

> *32. I am using CPAP for sleep apnea and getting restful sleep. Do I still need to lose weight (if I am overweight)?*

Yes. Weight loss is probably the most natural way of treating sleep apnea—no gadgets, no surgery, no drugs. Losing weight may result in needing less pressure on your CPAP unit, making it easier to tolerate. Sometimes, after losing enough weight, you may not need CPAP at all. Besides, losing weight will help you in other ways by making you more mobile and less prone to high blood pressure, heart disease, and even some types of arthritis.

> *33. I have been advised to use CPAP, but even after many weeks, I have not got used to it. What can I do?*

People differ in their ability to adapt to CPAP. Some take to it right away, while others take weeks or even months.

Even if you are not able to use it all night or every night, it is likely that with persistence, you will get more used to it. You may be able to make some adjustments to your unit. Increasing the so-called ramp time may allow you to fall asleep with a lower pressure, which increases after you are asleep. You could also try different levels of humidity—most units now come with a built-in heated humidifier. A different mask may also be more comfortable. Contact your CPAP supplier if you need help with these matters.

> *34. I have tried all the above suggestions but still can't get used to the CPAP machine. What are my other options?*

If the matter is not resolved, you may need to contact your healthcare provider for advice. Sometimes the pressure setting on the unit might need adjustment or a different type of unit with special features such as "auto-CPAP" may be required. This is a special unit that self-adjusts the pressure based on a built-in program. Sometimes, problems like nasal obstruction may require treatment before you can use CPAP comfortably.

As a last resort, you may have to switch from CPAP to a completely different form of treatment for your apnea. However, you should do so only with the knowledge and approval of your healthcare provider, since CPAP is the best treatment for sleep apnea, especially if it is severe.

35. I have been using CPAP for several weeks, but my sleepiness and fatigue are no better. What is the reason?

One reason may be that you have not yet adapted to CPAP. Sometimes this can take several weeks. You may not be using CPAP for long enough each night—some people remove the mask at night without realizing it. Another reason may be that the pressure set on your CPAP unit may need adjustment—check with your CPAP supplier or healthcare provider.

If you are using CPAP at the appropriate settings as recommended, but without any benefit, you may need to be reassessed. You may even be able to identify some problems yourself since you know your life better than anyone else. Remember that sleepiness and fatigue can be due to many reasons, not just sleep apnea. Factors such as insufficient sleep, poor sleeping routine and habits, insomnia, shift work, etc., can all produce these symptoms.

Treatment involves dealing with those issues that are causing the problem. For example, if you are depriving yourself of sleep by sleeping late and getting up early, the answer may be to try and get more hours of sleep, though this may not be easy with today's busy (and therefore sleep-deprived) lifestyle.

36. Can I go on vacation without my CPAP unit?

CPAP works by getting around a mechanical problem, which is intermittent blockage of the upper air passage. It cannot work when it is not being used. Not using it while on vacation will result in the return of your sleep apnea, not to mention that your snoring may disturb others (who wants to be sleepy and tired on vacation?).

The sensible thing to do is to use CPAP every time you sleep, whether you are on vacation or not. This is obviously more important if your apnea is severe.

By the way, never check in your CPAP unit when you fly—it may get lost or damaged, and you may need it either during the flight or shortly afterward. Take in on board with you (check with the airline if you need a note from your healthcare provider for this).

37. What are the problems one faces when using CPAP?

Some people notice discomfort from nasal congestion or drying, or skin irritation from the mask. Some people feel claustrophobic while trying to use the mask. These effects can be reduced or eliminated by proper fitting of the mask and adjusting the humidity (newer CPAP units come with a built-in humidifier). Occasionally, the air from the unit, being under slight pressure, can enter the stomach and cause a bloated feeling—this can be reduced by having the pressure turned down. Rare instances of ear or sinus infections have also been noted.

38. Can CPAP help me lose weight?

Although it is not a weight-loss method, CPAP can indirectly produce weight loss. When sleep apnea is treated with CPAP, it can be very effective in improving sleepiness and lethargy, making it easier to exercise and burn off calories. As a result, some people find it easier to lose weight while using CPAP, which in turn improves the severity of the sleep apnea (Figure 6). However, individual results with CPAP vary, and weight loss is not guaranteed just by using CPAP.

39. I am using CPAP. Are there any long-term side effects I should worry about?

In almost three decades of use, CPAP has helped millions of people with sleep apnea get restful sleep. CPAP has also resulted in tremendous benefits in terms of reduced risk of certain medical conditions. Remarkably, no significant long-term adverse side effects have been noted.

Some people think they will get "hooked" on CPAP. This is not true—unless they mean they get such good sleep with it that they do not want to give it up!

40. I am on oxygen at night for a lung condition. Can I stop using oxygen when I start using CPAP?

Probably not. CPAP simply keeps your upper air passage open so that you can breathe through it. It does not change the lung or heart condition for which the oxygen was ordered in the first place. When you start using CPAP, the oxygen can be channeled through a port on the CPAP mask.

Whether or not you need oxygen with CPAP can be checked with overnight pulse oximetry (see chapter 5)—for this you need to see your healthcare provider.

41. Can I use someone else's CPAP unit?

Generally, this is not recommended. Firstly, the pressure setting on someone else's unit may be different from what you need: one "size" does not fit all. Secondly, in the interest of personal hygiene, you should probably have your own mask and headgear rather than use someone else's (which would have to be really clean before you use it anyway). A borrowed mask is also less likely to fit properly. Lastly, you should not use anyone else's medical equipment if that person needs it.

If you have no choice and have to use someone else's CPAP unit, you should make sure the abovementioned factors are addressed, particularly regarding appropriate pressure setting, mask hygiene, and fitting.

42. How useful are commercially available nasal strips and specially designed pillows for sleep apnea?

These products help to reduce snoring. Nasal strips work by increasing the caliber of the nasal passages. However, the cause of sleep apnea is usually blockage in the throat area (pharynx), which is not changed by nasal strips, so they cannot really be expected to work for sleep apnea unless it is mild, and nasal obstruction is playing a role. Special pillows are supposed to work by supporting the neck in certain positions or by preventing the sleeper from rolling over on his or her back. Again, this may help with snoring but not necessarily with sleep apnea unless it is mild or positional (chapter 7).

These items have not been properly tested for sleep apnea. However, they are relatively inexpensive and there is probably no harm in trying them first, provided the apnea is mild and snoring is the main problem.

43. *I use a mouth guard for teeth grinding. Will this also work for snoring or sleep apnea?*

Not necessarily. The devices recommended for teeth grinding are usually designed to simply prevent the teeth from being damaged by grinding. Oral appliances for sleep apnea are designed to either move your jaw forward or to reposition the tongue, thereby increasing the space through which you can breathe.

If you are seriously considering an oral appliance for snoring or sleep apnea, contact a dentist or denturist trained in the use of such devices. Remember that these devices are generally less effective than CPAP, especially if the apnea is severe.

44. *I had surgery (UPPP) for snoring and sleep apnea. Should I be checked to see if the apnea is gone?*

Ideally, yes. A sleep study, or at least some form of home study, can be arranged a few months after UPPP (to allow time to heal). This is obviously more important if the surgery was done for severe apnea and for some reason you could not have CPAP, since the operation may not take away all of the apnea. However, the final decision about how you are evaluated after surgery will have to be made in consultation with your healthcare provider after taking into account your individual circumstances.

45. *Can oxygen be used to treat sleep apnea?*

OSA is caused by obstruction of the upper air passage. Giving oxygen by itself in this condition will not open up the passage, so oxygen by itself is unlikely to help. However, it may help if the oxygen level remains low even after using treatment such as CPAP.

Oxygen can have good and bad effects in sleep apnea. It can improve the oxygen level, particularly if it is used as described above, but it can sometimes prolong the apneas. Checking the oxygen level at night with overnight pulse oximetry should be considered if oxygen is used.

Oxygen by itself has occasionally been used for central sleep apnea, where obstruction is not the issue.

Bibliography

Dickens C. *The Posthumous Papers of the Pickwick Club*. Chapman & Hall, 1837.

Dement WC. *The Sleepwatchers*. 2nd ed. Nychthemeron Press, 1996.

Mazzagatti FA, Lebowitz LC, Schugler NW. *Respiratory Care Pearls*. Hanley & Belfus Inc., 1997.

Chokroverty S. *Clinical Companion to Sleep Disorders Medicine*. 2nd ed. Butterworth-Heinemann, 2000.

Stevens DR. *Sleep Medicine Secrets*. Hanley & Belfus Inc., 2004.

Hirshkowitz M, Smith PB. *Sleep Disorders for Dummies*. Wiley Publishing Inc., 2004.

Chokroverty S, Thomas RJ, Bhatt M. *Atlas of Sleep Medicine*. Elsevier Inc., 2005.

Hensrud DD, ed. *Mayo Clinic Healthy Weight for Everybody*. 1st ed. Mayo Foundation for Medical Education and Research, 2005.

Kryger MH, Roth T, Dement WC. *Principles and Practice of Sleep Medicine*. 4th ed. WB Saunders Co., 2005.

Bordow RA, Reis AL, Morris TA, eds. *Manual of Clinical Problems in Pulmonary Medicine*. 6th ed. Lippincott Williams & Wilkins, 2005.

Avidan AY, Zee PH. *Handbook of Sleep Medicine.* Lippincott Williams & Wilkins, 2006.

Fleetham J, Ayas N, Bradley D, Ferguson K, Fitzpatick M, George C, et al. *Canadian Thoracic Society guidelines: diagnosis and treatment of sleep disordered breathing in adults.* Can Resp J 2006;13(7)387-92.

Pagel JS, Pandi-Perumal SR, eds. *Primary Care Sleep Medicine.* Humana Press Inc., 2007.

Abrams B. *The Perils of Sleep Apnea—An Undiagnosed Epidemic—A Layman's Perspective.* iUniverse, 2007.

Pascualy R. *Snoring and Sleep Apnea—Sleep Well, Feel Better.* 4th ed. Demos Medical Publishing, 2008.

Soparkar G. *Questions and Answers in Sleep Apnea (An Internist's Perspective).* Xlibris, 2009.

American Sleep Apnea Association: *www.sleepapnea.org.*

National Sleep Foundation: *www.sleepfoundation.org.*

Index

65207508R00053

Made in the USA
Middletown, DE
23 February 2018